LAUGHTER, SEX, VEGETABLES & FISH

10 Secrets of Long Living People

DR JOHN TICKELL

Published by
Crown Content
A.C.N. 096 393 636
A.B.N. 37 096 393 636
Level 1, 141 Capel Street
North Melbourne Vic. 3051
Telephone: (03) 9329 9800
Fax: (03) 9329 9698

Dr John Tickell
PO Box 1431
Noosa Heads Qld 4567
Telephone: (07) 5474 8960
Email: drjohntickell@drjohntickell.com
Website: www.drjohntickell.com

The National Library of Australia
Cataloguing-in-Publication entry:

Tickell, John.
  The 10 secrets of long living people : laughter, sex, vegetables & fish.

  ISBN 1 86350 345 5

  1. Stress magagement - Popular works. 2. Stress (Psychology) -
  Popular works. 3. Self-care, Health. 4. Longevity - Nutritional aspects -
  Popular works. I. Title. II. Title : Ten secrets of long living people.

155.9042

Cover & Page Design: Ben Graham

Printed in Australia by McPherson's Printing Group.

CONTENTS

FOREWORD

T he world is full of specialists, technical experts and people who love to complicate things.

As a Medical Doctor, I have grown up in an environment where, by nature, things do get complicated. The human machine is an incredible conglomerate of bits and pieces and amazing chemical reactions.

If I have any ability at all, it is the ability to simplify complicated things.

There is a minefield of misinformation out there which definitely confuses us in the ways of eating, exercising and getting our brains into gear.

As a prescriber of exercise, a self-taught nutritionist and an amateur psychologist, I can beat the hell out of almost every author on these topics. That is simply because of my experience with real people in the land of general practice, consulting with thousands of patients, delivering their babies, sharing their joys and sorrows - in the land of business, consulting with the captains of industry and coal miners alike - in the land of sport, treating the elite and the also-rans.

So I offer you the ultimate personal 'How To' book....

And it works!

A CASE IN POINT

In a busy general practice, it became not only obvious over the years, but concerning, that patients tended to fall into two distinct groups.

On the one hand, a patient with a surgical emergency, a bacterial infection or injury as a result of a trauma/accident such as a broken bone can be helped immediately by the 'good old Doc'.

On the other hand, patients with lifestyle diseases such as most heart disease, various forms of arthritis, the most common cancers and most other ailments, are in a different basket.

These problems do not have a single cause. The causative and precipitating factors are multiple and in most cases we mumble about genetics and so on, but perhaps the real culprits are the lousy food we eat, the inactivity, the environmental pollutants and how unhappy and dissatisfied we are?

It is difficult to alter the path of someone's life in seven to 10 minutes in a doctor's office, and this was apparent to me as I drifted into a situation where I was spending an hour or an hour and a half with each person.

While it may border on the unethical to fully quote the various cases of patients who have turned their lives around, I have no hesitation in jotting down for your interest portions of a few of the amazing number of letters that come my way.

"I still have you to thank for being here today - no doubt about that!" P.G.S., Petersham.

"Your book was devoured in one sitting, then absorbed over a number of readings. My current lifestyle is a constant talking point - the new me. I altered my pattern of exercise when you told me swimming was not going to help reduce my weight. I will never go on a diet again. In four months I have lost 19 kg! Dr John, I am indebted to you for the gift you gave me. I will have a longer, happier life." P.C., Geelong.

"I have the usual collection of diet books. Your advice is truly a miracle. With absolutely no pain, I have lost 6kg of flab and my husband has lost 13kg and looks just beautiful! I have a power now, l am in control, and other people want that power!" V.K., Wahroonga.

"Your presentation was riveting. I purchased your book and video program. I am a 34-year-old woman who has been smoking for many years. I've done it - I've given them up - I've actually done it! I am becoming more intelligent every day and feeling fantastic! Thank-you again." J.N., Salisbury Heights.

"I walked out of the Tennis Centre and the words were ringing in my ears: "It is impossible to be intelligent and smoke at the same time." I threw them in the bin and haven't touched one since." A.G., Essendon.

"Outstanding. Please send 60 books, one for each of my staff. I can't let this opportunity pass." V.H., Honolulu.

"Over the years I have listened to many presentations in Australia and overseas. Without doubt, the highlight of the Congress. My wife and I thank you. Each time we fly over Coolum in future we will give you a warm salute." D.R., Gold Coast.

"I have been telling my friends that you and I can take half the credit each for turning my life around. Also, I have lost 15 kg without trying. I can't believe it was so simple, so sensible." H.K., Mt Eliza.

"Thank-you. I want to tell you today I am 68, I have beaten bowel cancer, I have a 33-year-old wife and feel 45!!" Dr K.G.M., Albany.

"All I want is another video, quickly - my previous one is worn out with use from my patients." Dr R.S., Te Aroha.

"Heartiest congratulations on your video The Stress of Success. *I'm a medical adviser to one of the biggest banks in the country and have recommended your presentation for the executive staff health program."* Dr D.H., Sydney.

"What your 'moderation in everything' approach has done for me is unbelievable." T.S., Singapore.

"My sister sent me your book from Sydney. She said it would fix everything. It has. Many thanks." S.W., London, UK.

THE THIRD THIRD OF MANAGEMENT SKILLS

W hat happened to the first two?

Don't worry about it. I thought I'd start with the third third and cover the other two later.

You're getting uptight already. Just settle down and leave it to me. It's my book, OK?

A while back, I was fortunate to meet the man who probably 'invented' the word stress - an Austrian-born Canadian professor called Hans Selye.

I think he might have died drinking champagne on a dance floor when he was getting on towards 90.

He used to tell me that people didn't really understand the word stress.

People still stay to me, "Listen mate, I'm under stress" and I say, "But there's no stress out there to be under, because stress is in here ... stress is an internal phenomenon."

What's out there is called PRESSURE ... the stressor ... pressure. If you put the same pressure in front of six people, how come you get six different stress responses? Because the individual chooses ... that's how come. Same pressure - different response.

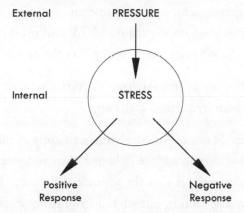

Now let's take person No. 1 in the line-up and they consider this pressure and they feel good about it because their attitudes are pretty good and they say, "Great, I'm going to respond well to this. I'm going to win for me, for my group, my family, my company, my organisation." To the person who takes that attitude, that pressure is a challenge to stimulate positive action, and they generally have a positive response and feel good about it because the human body loves a positive response.

There is no down side to this stuff, it's brilliant.

What about person No. 2, who is faced with exactly the same pressure?

Person No.1 is thriving on this pressure, so why does Person No. 2 have a negative reaction? Why?

Well it's in your heart and it's in your mind. It's an attitude and it's a feeling.

The city I come from down under is Melbourne, Australia. We have some lovely fine weather and some not so fine weather, and yet you turn to the weather forecast in Melbourne on an ordinary day and do you know what they say on the radio and TV and print in the paper? - 'partly cloudy'. So why not 'partly sunny'? It's the same thing, isn't it?

I know of no bureau of meteorology in Australia with a computer forecast of partly sunny ... there aren't any.

Yet, in the United States of America, you get a copy of the newspaper *USA Today*, flip it over to see the coloured map and you read all the 'partly sunny' forecasts - is that the attitude difference? It's the same picture, blue sky and clouds, but what do you really want to see, and what do you really want to happen?

(My dad was a meteorologist. He said to me that a meteorologist was someone who could look into a girl's eyes and tell whether...)

The great thing about a positive attitude is that we positive creatures are definitely in the minority. There are a lot fewer of us because the great majority of people are negative thinkers, so that means there is a lot more room for us to move and manoeuvre. The ball park on our side is wide open.

Imagine if everyone saw the silver lining in the clouds and imagine if everyone saw the opportunity in adversity - it would be an awful crush.

On the positive side of the ledger, there is so much space to spread your wings. Try it sometime - the freedom feels so good.

Smile a little and move over this side.

People say, "Yeah ... but what about tough times?" Well, what about them? I think tough times are great because very few genuine winners ever come out of good times. Remember the last boom? The winners that come out of boom times are usually fleeting winners - here today, gone tomorrow. It's the tough times when genuine winners are born. That's what is so good about tough times. Remember, the pressures on everybody are the same, and it's your choice whether you have positive responses or chronic negative responses. *It is your choice.*

There is another alternative - no response at all. This is what we call the vegetable or blank response - for people living in a vacuum who never do anything or get anywhere. Sometimes this response can be quite valuable.

I'll give you a few tips later about how to learn to love pressure.

You might get away with a certain amount of negative response in your 20s and early 30s but if you are in your late 30s and into the Dangerous Decade (44 to 54) and you pile the negative responses on top of one another, what are you doing? You are destroying your immune system; you are cutting yourself to bits; your resistance is dropping away.

People say to me, "What do you mean; what's the immune system?"

You know what that is ... the immune system is the thing inside you that decides if you get a head cold or influenza next week. The immune system is the thing that decides to a large extent whether you get cancer in five or eight years ... and you personally have enormous control over your immune system. If you want to get a head cold next week, if you don't want to get a head cold next week ... it's up to you, to a large extent.

"That's rubbish!" they say.

It's not rubbish. If you walk down the street with 100 people and someone with the worst influenza in the world coughs all over the entire 100 people, how come only 20 or 25 catch the influenza? They are the ones with the worst resistance at the time, the downers, the miserable people, and the ones who aren't coping very well.

If you get a dripping nose and you go straight to bed and call in sick, how long is your problem going to last? Maybe seven or eight days.

If you get a dripping nose and the first time you actually notice this is when it's dripping on the papers on your desk, and you're excited about the project on your desk, it won't last eight days - maybe two or four days.

This is because the dripping nose is a minor event, not a major event, and you've been able to put that little dripping nose in a box in a corner of your brain. It isn't a big deal, just a little deal (minor irritation). There is control here. We'll discuss it later.

I'll say it again. Stress in internal - it is your choice what you do with it.

There, I've said it again.

Next I'm going to tell you about pressure. I know all about pressure because I'm an expert on pressure.

I've had thousands of clients with pressure. I developed a $150 million resort without any money - that's pressure - and besides, I have five kids. Pressure, pressure and more pressure.

This might sound serious and I apologise for that, but in fact pressure is serious enough to have a chapter named after it.

PRESSURE

P ressure is incredible stuff. It is both frightening and exciting. In short bursts it is stimulating. In long, drawn-out doses, it is soul-destroying.

When times are good we put ourselves under tremendous pressure to succeed, and when times are lousy we put ourselves under tremendous pressure not to fail. It all comes back to the human ego and the human ego is an almighty thing.

We hate to be talked of as a failure, to be written about as a failure, to be seen as a failure. Failure does not sit well with Western living and the success expected of people living the Western life.

Failure is not well tolerated.

I believe my book can help you. I will discuss with you the effects of pressure; how to deal with it; how to use it for your benefit; how to run away from it; and, most important of all, how to learn to love it.

LIFE

Life is about ego, achievement, self-esteem, sunshine, laughter, hugging, negotiating, doing things for other people and looking forward to things.

Life is about please and thank you and doing your best.

If your kids don't say please and thank you and don't have respect for their fellow human beings, then you haven't brought them up very well.

Life is all about friends too.

Having someone to talk to is a very powerful medicine. Many studies show the value of a close friend, a confidant, a support group.

The immune system is just so much stronger; it is too real to ignore.

HOW MUCH,
HOW MANY?

The movies and the books used to say, 'greed is good'. So greed *was* good, but not now?

Nevertheless, the basis of greed was counting. To be a 'success' in a 'civilised country' one needed to surround oneself with numbers - the how much and how many of life.

But counting is also a part of achievement (especially in the younger years) and while greed may not be good any more, achievement *is good* and if you need to count to achieve, then so be it.

How many goals did you score? How many runs did you make? How many operas did you sing at? How many reports did you type?

And the corporations have big scoreboards with dollars all over them - count, count, count. If counting is a measure of achievement, then that is good, but everything is relative, isn't it?

One thing to one person is something else to someone else.

PERSONALITIES

A factor that plays an enormous part in the process of success or failure, and whether you make it to the top and whether you stay there, is the personality of the person and the type of behaviour they display.

You have heard of the Type A person.

Type A people are generally considered ambitious. They are fast-moving creatures; they often get aggressive when things slow down; they tap their pen on the table; their knee jiggles under the desk; and their foot goes up and down because things just aren't going fast enough for them.

Type As tend to hate queues and they especially hate red traffic lights - they go down several side streets and get there at the same time, but at least they were doing something.

The As might have lunch at their desk, but they have phones hanging off their heads, piles of paper on the desk, files on the floor, and organised disorganisation.

Type A males always push the flush button on the toilet way before they finish peeing.

Type A people are irritated by other people who talk really slowly. The Type A tends to lean over the desk and at the first opportunity interrupts the other person, finishing the sentence for them, just to get things going faster.

Type As are considered good at business and achieve success more quickly than others.

If you want something done then give it to a Type A person because it will be done - it will be slotted somewhere in a busy day.

Nevertheless, people with Type A behaviour may run higher risks in the health stakes.

Type Bs, on the other hand, are more laid back about life - the "she'll be right mate" people.

Type B behaviour people feel that no problem is a great problem; it will probably fix itself, so really what's the hassle?

These Type Bs tend to sit back on their chairs in meetings while Type As are leaning forward.

Type Bs tend to be less successful in the way that the Western system measures success but on the positive side they tend to live a long time!

Another behaviour type that I shall refer to as Type C is a real worry. I am concerned about people who display C Type behaviour because of the risks these people run.

Type C persons can often fool you because they look like they are handling the world pretty well. They tend to have a bland expression on their face and they sit upright on the chair rather than forward or backward, but C Types are suppressing feelings. All the pressures, fears, jealousies, problems, they are internalising - they stew on them and they never get things off their chest and discuss them openly with others.

Let's look at my opinions regarding the health risks of these three behaviour types.

Type As tend to run higher risks for the vascular diseases — that is the heart attacks and strokes. I will qualify that statement in a little while, but take that as a generalisation.

Type Bs don't risk much at all, and Type Cs run higher risks of internal diseases such as cancers.

People naturally react and tell me that I can't prove this and I am the first to agree because it is impossible to put people on a scale and measure their behaviour types and responses to certain conditions over a period of time. It is a simple matter to measure cholesterol or a blood pressure, but very difficult to measure behaviour types or stress responses and categorise them.

Then again, a cholesterol of 180 (4.5) is no guarantee of long life, because there is no account taken of the unmeasurable factors about which I am talking.

Of course, this is one of the problems with Western medicine, isn't it? Western medicine depends on *absolute proof* before it accepts anything.

Nevertheless, I can type a person's behaviour by merely talking to them for a few minutes, then watching them for a few more.

But behaviour is a fluid thing and you can change behaviour and your reactions if you want to.

One of the interesting characteristics of some A behaviour males is that their typical A behaviour disappears when they go home, and they go way across to the brooding C Type, saying nothing, discussing nothing. This is particularly rough on the spouse who is expected to deal with this extrovert turned grumpy introvert. It can destroy relationships if you're not careful.

You are born with a personality - that is you are given one to start with - that's the genetic influence. Then your parents have about four or five years to mould your personality environmentally. Obviously, that's very scary from the parents' point of view because the first five years are definitely the formative years when children learn to behave the way they do.

Basically, after five years the parents lose their influence over kids' personalities or behaviour types and the school environment gets the next go. Then the business houses grab you and in Western countries tend to force behaviour to the Type A end of the scale.

Is that bad? Not necessarily, because some Type A people do survive the rat race.

HOW TYPE A
MANIACS SURVIVE

Some Type A people do survive the rat race and the qualification on the statement that I made before about Type As and the risks they run is this:

If Type A maniacs wish to survive, they need some special qualities.

QUALITY NO. 1 - you must retain or relearn the process of dropping back one slot and become a B Type behaviour person for three minutes or three hours or three days, now and again, as the situation demands.

QUALITY NO. 2 - Type As must have the ability to listen to themselves and become aware of the warning signs that the body throws up - the little cracks that appear. If you don't take notice of these warning signs and act upon them, then you are merely waiting for the *final event,* the heart attack, the stroke, the diabetes, the burst ulcer, etc. The final event is obviously far too late.

QUALITY NO. 3 - Lack of hostility. Perhaps the major difference between Type As who survive and Type As who destroy themselves is this hostility streak which seems to develop in many Type A persons as life goes on.

The hostile As start to become irritable and become annoyed by just about anything - air conditioners, people, little noises, clocks, flies, kids, whatever ... things that don't need to annoy you.

Hostile people start to lose friends and they may end up with a pile of money, but so what? Remember that life is all about friends too. If you haven't got any friends, you've got nothing.

So what's the best behaviour type to have? I mean it's great to be a B Type but they don't climb many corporate ladders or in fact ladders of any sort. C Types do but they harm themselves in the process. So what is best?

I think the ideal is to swing between the A and B behaviour types.

If fact, I don't think - I know!

When you are in the pressure cooker, run hard and keep your eye on the ball, but when you are out of the pressure cooker, learn how to switch *off* and laugh and dream a little.

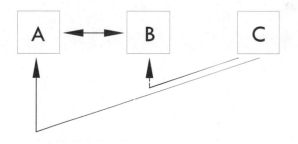

SHOULD I DIE FEELING GOOD OR FEELING BAD?

If you choose to live in a Western country, you have a 10% chance of dying of old age feeling good.

One in 10 of us is going to live through until we are 87 or 94 or 97, then we'll go to bed one night, and the next morning we'll be dead - and we won't have died of anything. People say, "Well that's no good, you have to die of something", but you don't you know. I mean some people literally die when they've finished living, and the common example of that is the spouse who dies six to eight months after the other spouse. No disease - they have just lost the will to live. They've lost that little spark, that ambition, that drive, that goal that is always so necessary in life.

"I'm looking forward to retirement; I'm retiring in two or three years you know." That's fine, but you can't fish forever and unless you do have that little spark you'll shrivel up.

How many people three years after they've retired are totally ineffective and almost, if not, dead? They are just not being fair to themselves.

So 10% of us get by, and the next 10% of us die of bad luck, and you can't help bad luck. That's 20%. The other 80% of us (that's four out of five) are going to kill ourselves prematurely and way ahead of time.

And, of course, most people consider that they're fine - it's the two people either side of them who are in trouble.

If you are going to kill yourself there are some fantastic new diseases from which to choose - diseases which have moved rapidly up the hit parade in the past few decades.

These degenerative diseases - the heart disease, the heart attacks, the strokes, the sugar diabetes, the kidney problems, the bowel problems, the anxiety neuroses and many of the cancers - have taken over from the diseases of the early 20th century which killed us in our youth, such as the infectious diseases - typhoid, cholera, polio and tuberculosis.

It's time you met George.

George is an executive acquaintance of mine, who used to be a non believer (a total sceptic). Then George was forced to attend one of my seminars and he became a half believer (mild sceptic) after a few things actually stuck in his mind and made sense.

So at this stage George says to me, "Well that's fine, but you can't help cancer - cancer is bad luck."

I think the latest research tends to show that 70% or more of cancers have very little to do with bad luck - they're more likely to be our fault.

Look at the cancer profiles in men and women in Western countries. Males first. The two big cancer killers in males are obviously lung cancer and colon cancer (that's bowel cancer). Add those two together and you have almost half the cancer deaths in males and people say it's bad luck? Prostate cancer statistics have also become significant.

Let's look more closely at this.

Around 3% to 5% of males who die of lung cancer don't smoke, and the other 95% or so do smoke or did smoke. That's called 'A RISK'. Interesting isn't it?

I mean, think of the risks associated with Western living. Life's full of risks, but if you are taking this particular risk, then have a *really* hard look.

There are two relevant statements regarding cigarette smoking.

STATEMENT NO. I

IT IS IMPOSSIBLE TO BE INTELLIGENT AND SMOKE AT THE SAME TIME.

There's an exception, there's always an exception; every rule has an exception. If it's 1.15 in the morning and you're in a bar and you are half boozed and you've had a few too many drinks and you pull out a big fat cigar and stick it in your face, then light it and take a puff - that's fine isn't it? - because you're stupid at 1.15 in the morning.

But it's hard to do it to yourself when you wake up to the cold, hard light of day. Very hard to do it to yourself, especially if you are fair dinkum.

STATEMENT NO. 2

THE AVERAGE SMOKER SMOKES 20 CIGARETTES A DAY FOR 35 YEARS. THAT'S 250,000 CIGARETTES.

Now that's not a group, that's each average smoker - 250,000 of the little buggers, and there's 10 puffs in every cigarette.

So that's 2.5 million times that crap is going through this brilliant computer called the human system. If you could find a computer this good (and you can't), would you stand alongside it blowing all that smoke through it? You'd stuff it up, wouldn't you?

People do it to themselves. Unbelievable, isn't it?

Unbelievable!

PS: If your lungs were on the outside (instead of the inside), where you could actually see them, no-one - but no-one - would smoke.

THE BIG ONE
IN WOMEN

B reast cancer is the big one in women.

The biggest killer in men under 60 in Western countries is heart attack, which is fairly obvious, but the biggest killer in women under 60 is breast cancer. Every year, thousands and thousands of women under 60 die of breast cancer and very few should. It's just not fair. Much of the problem is a lack of awareness and lack of prevention.

Any woman who does not have a breast check and a smear check (on the cervix, that's the neck of the womb) every couple of years after they've moved into their 20s, is crazy. If you don't do that, you are playing Russian Roulette, because these are often curable diseases in their early stages.

Breast cancer seems to be a disease of Western countries - the eating, the pressure, the inactivity. The incidence in countries where women live a simple existence and eat simple foods is quite low.

But overall now, the biggest cancer in Western countries is bowel cancer. It's moved to the top of the pops when you add men and women together.

It is interesting that lung cancer statistics in middle-aged males seem to show a decline in the disease in this group, but middle-aged women still show an increase in the figures (for obvious reasons) and the kids fill the gaps.

Middle-aged males are giving up smoking more readily than women.

It doesn't matter if you smoke when you're 18, does it? I mean, it's 30 to 40 years before anything happens or it affects you.

Do you know how many 18-year-olds smoke? - up to 40% - that's a hell of a lot.

Once they move up to about 30 years old, the percentage of smokers comes back to the national average - 30% or a little less - still unbelievable! Even more adults smoke in Asia and Europe because the cigarette companies have to make money somehow. Who are the people at 30 who are still smoking? Generally the kids who were growing up in smoking environments.

It doesn't matter whether your child hates or loves you, they do tend to copy. They often revert to copying in later life what happened in those first few years. And if you as a parent sat there and ate lots of vegetables for the first five years of the child's life, the child would think that is normal behaviour. If you grew up with mainly meats and cheeses and that's what you ate in front of your child, the child would think that's normal. If you're smoking, both parents especially, then that is accepted as normal. Pretty simple. Eh?

WHAT TAKES FOUR MINUTES IN THE MORNING?

Bowel cancer has now moved to the No. 1 position in most 'civilised' countries.

George says, "Well that is bad luck."

But wait just a moment. Have a look at the mechanics of the intestines. Let's say this tube is your intestines. Up the top is the wide end - it's called your mouth - and down there is the other end.

MOUTH

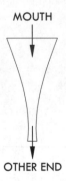

OTHER END

Now the emptying time of this tube (the transit time) is the time it takes the toxic products and poisons - all that stuff in the bowel - to move from one end to the other. The transit time seems to be in inverse proportion (this means upside down) to your risk of getting low bowel diseases - like the haemorrhoids, the piles, the diverticulitis, the ulcers, the bowel cancers. So, basically, the slower the stuff moves through the pipe, the higher the risk of bowel disease.

And do you know that most people deliberately go out of their way to slow down the emptying time of this pipe? And the best way to deliberately do this is to refuse point blank to eat that meal called breakfast.

Breakfast used to be two words - break fast.

And break fast breaks a 17-hour fast between dinner last night and lunch today. Type A people who are in a dreadful hurry have now squeezed up the two words break fast into one word, which is a lot quicker to say ... breakfast.

Breakfast does break a 17-hour fast and it is particularly important for the non-copers among us, especially those who are rolling along into that Dangerous Decade - the decade from 44 to 54 when responsible people under tremendous pressure start to fall to bits.

Things fall out, things fall off, things go into spasm, and they never recognise this as part of the non-coping syndrome.

So most of the non-copers eat all their food in seven hours (between 1 pm and 8 pm) and stuff all (almost nothing) for the next 17 hours except a coffee and a cigarette in the morning to kick start the motor.

Now that's just ridiculous. If you had half a brain you *would* get up four minutes earlier wouldn't you? You *would* sit at a table and you *would* stick some roughage in the top of that pipe in the morning to get things going.

Roughage is fibre and fibre is in food. It's the indigestible part of food that goes right on through, acting as both a stimulant and sponge. Fibre is only in plant foods. It is in vegetables, and fresh fruits (not as much in stewed fruit because a lot of it has been broken down), and there's fibre in grains, breads, and cereals. So fibre at breakfast time means some wholegrain bread and/or a bowl of grain cereal or porridge, some chopped up banana or other fruits and some low-fat milk.

George says, "Hey, wait a minute, we have real full cream milk at our house", and I say, "What do you mean?"

"Cow's milk."

Good for cows, not so good for humans - it is very fatty stuff.

So why do you need full cream milk?

"Well, the kids need it", and I say, "Why?" and George says, "Well ... they just do because *they* said."

Now hang on, listen ... not so long ago when I was a real doctor seeing sick people, and some who thought they were sick, I was also a part-time obstetrician. I delivered hundreds of babies before I hung up my gloves.

Most of the women involved in these child births breast-fed their babies and how brilliantly do babies go on human breast milk? They thrive on the stuff, it pumps up the immune system, and human breast milk has a lot less saturated fat than cow's milk. So why do kids need cow's milk? - because *they* said? I mean, lower fat milks, for example, have usually at least the same amount of protein and more calcium. Just less fat.

The cereals.

If you are going to eat packaged cereals, you have to be careful. The food labelling laws in the United States are pretty good, but the food labelling laws in most other Western countries aren't so good. So read the box - some of the cereals are so bad it would be better to eat the box, because there's more roughage in the cardboard.

Be wary of the excess sugars, refined products and coconut or coconut oils which are a bit fanciful in so-called health cereals - we'll talk about it later. It takes four minutes a day to reduce your risk of developing the biggest cancer in the Western world, so why wouldn't you do it?

Too busy? Type A maniac? Four lousy minutes - not a bad idea - and this is not fanatical stuff. I personally worry about fanatics because fanatics are so intense about things they often turn other people off whatever they are fanatical about. Fanatics can become socially unacceptable, like fanatical exercisers.

Now if it's a gold medal you're striving for, then pain and sweat are definitely necessary. If it's just life you're after, then take it a little easier.

I've been in the management skills business for 20 years or more and I have dealt with literally thousands and thousands of executives, sales people and managers, and the experience has taught me many things. It can all be summed up in my great motto:

MODERATION IN ALL THINGS.

The 20 years have also shown me four things that you can potentially use to excess and I assure you that a lot of research has gone into this. The four excesses are:

LAUGHTER - that's a *big* one.

SEX - although there's some doubt about that right now ... a lot of doubt indeed.

VEGETABLES and

FISH

So the motto now reads

MODERATION IN ALL THINGS ... EXCEPT LAUGHTER, SEX, VEGETABLES AND FISH.

No particular order, and not all together - it makes one hell of a mess!

Now the reasons you can overuse these things.

LAUGHTER AND SEX are the best two stress cycle breakers known to the human system. We are not sure whether they are No. 1 and No. 2 or No. 2 and No. 1. But if they come together you are getting old.

VEGETABLES form the basis of the food groups eaten by the races of people in this world who live the longest and feel the best. There is no argument here. We can look at these people and they're 75, they're 80, and they look like we do when we are 55 or 65.

So what's the difference? One big difference is the amount of plant food these people consume.

FISH. The fish story is very impressive. We know from the research that races of people who eat at least two meals of fish a week have an incidence of heart attack and stroke way lower than Western populations because fish oils seem to protect arteries.

Maybe you can help by taking fish oil capsules, but you sure as hell can by eating real fish. The deep sea and cold water fish seem to be the best - tuna, mackerel, herrings, sardines, salmon.

ALTERNATIVE TO SEX

I have a very good friend who is a big downer on sex. We call her the Queen of the Celibates. I've talked and talked at length with this person about the subject and eventually we've come to an agreement.

If you want, YOU CAN REPLACE SEX WITH RICE.

It's not very comfortable, but it's very good for you.

THE WARNING SIGNS

W hat about those little warning signs of negative stress we mentioned before - the little cracks that appear one by one?

How do I know if the pressure is getting to me? I think I'm OK but am I kidding myself?

There's a heap of little warning signs and we'll go through them.

WARNING NO. 1 - MUSCLE SPASM.

This is a warning sign that people usually disregard. Muscle spasm takes different forms in different areas of the body and it's called various things - maybe a headache, a migraine, a pain in the neck. People sit at their desks and they're all hunched up. I say, "Relax." They say, "I am relaxed, but my neck's gone", and I go round the back and say, "No, your neck's still there."

It is just in spasm - your neck is screaming at you. It is saying please, please just jump out of the pressure cooker and become a B Type for three minutes ... just unwind ... just relax. Your body is telling you that, and if you don't listen to your body, you're crazy.

Muscle spasm a little lower down is chest pain. People think they are having a heart spasm or heart attack. Usually it is just a spasm of the muscles between the ribs because you are so tense. Your body once again is telling you something. Heart pain (angina) is usually not a sharp or stabbing pain but rather a tightness or pressure feeling, like someone tightening a huge rubber band around your chest or placing a heavy weight on it. Angina may also feel like indigestion that won't go away. The pain may radiate to your neck or arms. Obviously, if you are uncertain, you quickly get to hospital or call an ambulance.

Gut pain - that's acid pouring in your stomach. If acid pours into your stomach in major quantities in the middle of the night, then you wake up with gut pain. It may be just a transient pain, but if it lasts half an hour or an hour, what's possibly happening is that you could be developing a little crater ulcer - boy is that a warning!

People take pills and say it doesn't matter, another glass of milk, she'll be right mate. The body is pleading with you, saying please, just be a B Type for a day, or how about three days?

A common symptom of not coping in middle-aged males is lower back pain, and this is generally muscle spasm rather than a serious problem.

A great deal of adult diarrhoea has nothing to do with infection - it's spasm of the colon. People go to the doctor and the doctor says, "Well, that has a fancy name. It's called 'Irritable Bowel Syndrome' or 'Irritable Colon' or some type of colitis."

So what's the best treatment for this? Pills maybe. Maybe, but what about the other answer. Is there an alternative answer to this warning?

Unwind, relax ... the spasm may go.

These are the spasms and warnings that people build brick walls in front of. Don't build brick walls; treat them for what they are - warnings.

WARNING NO. 2 - THE STIMULANTS SYNDROME or the CATS SYNDROME.

What are the CATS?

Caffeine, Alcohol, Tobacco and Sugars refined and processed.

How much chemical stimulation do you need to survive?

How much caffeine, how much alcohol do you need - how much tobacco and nicotine do you need every day - how much refined and processed sugar do you need to survive? I'm not saying you are not allowed to use them at all. Don't get me wrong, the human body just loves a kick now and again.

My experience with thousands of executives has shown me the levels of stimulants that most people can get away with and still survive.

How much caffeine? Maybe up to two or three shots a day is OK. George says to me, "Now hang on ... I've heard you shouldn't drink coffee at all. It's no good for you, you know."

Well some people like the stuff - it gives them a kick. But if you use four, eight, 10, 12 cups a day then forget it. That's over the top. That's a *warning*.

If you have a coffee machine in your office and every time you are hassled you go straight to the machine and zap yourself with another dose of caffeine, then you're on the stimulant roller coaster. You're up there for 20 minutes after your shot of caffeine and then you come down, possibly not to normal but underground. You begin to get irritable, you get a bit depressed and you need another coffee, another cigarette, another cookie and you're up there again.

What's the alternative? Ever heard of a glass of iced water with a slice of lemon?... brilliant stuff.

Where's the iced water dispenser in the office? Water goes in the same cup, it's liquid, it goes in the same hole in your face and it tastes great.

Why do you want more than two or maximum three coffees a day?... you don't need it.

Alcohol.

People say, "Now hang on, this stuff is dangerous. You just can't drink alcohol - it's an addictive drug".

Some people cannot and must not touch alcohol at all. It is an absolute NO.

For those of us who are able to use alcohol, there are several points to consider.

If you lined up all the drugs in the world, nicotine would come at the worst end. Smoking cigarettes is probably the greatest expression of non-coping there is. There are bad drugs and not so bad drugs. If you look at alcohol as a drug, it seems to nudge into the not-so-bad end of the drug scale if used very carefully.

Note the positive features that alcohol can have on many human bodies.

The first two or three drinks relax you (the next 13 don't). While alcohol technically is a depressant, the first two or three drinks relax and stimulate you because they release or take the inhibitions away, which can be a good thing now and then.

Alcohol thins the blood which can be quite positive.

Alcohol pumps up the production of a chemical, the high-density lipo-protein, in the blood. It actually raises the level of these proteins and they scavenge cholesterol. They drag cholesterol out of the arteries and take it back to the liver, which is pretty clever, isn't it? So it's been shown that people who drink some alcohol may have a lower risk of heart disease. The other great thing about alcohol - if you have enough of the stuff, it can make ugly people look really beautiful!

But if you let it grab you, you're gone.

How much is the right amount?

My assessment (from the research) is that men can get away with up to 20-25 drinks a week and women somewhat less, providing everything else in your life is in place.

I'll tell you why women don't tolerate alcohol as well. The liver in women just doesn't work quite the same when it is metabolising the alcohol - it seems to happen more slowly.

On the flip side of that coin of course is the good news about women's hearts. They are smaller, more effective, and protected by female hormones - thus women's hearts tend to last seven or eight years longer than men's hearts.

But we are talking about alcohol here.

George asks, "What actually is a drink - a bottle, a jug or what?"

Well, a standard drink is 7 ounces of beer, 4 ounces of wine, or I ounce of Scotch or another spirit. So in a small bottle or stubby or can of beer, there are one-and-a-half to two drinks, and in a bottle of wine, around six drinks.

Men tell me they share a bottle of wine with their spouse in the evenings. Generally speaking, a shared bottle of wine between a man and a woman means the woman drinks one-and-a-half glasses and the man four-and-a-half glasses.

"But we shared it!"

We kid ourselves when it comes to how much we drink. In a bottle of Scotch there are 26 drinks - not two as some people count it. And people say, "I've gone off the Scotch mate, I'm only drinking wine", or, "But I've given up beer, it's fattening you know - I only drink spirits now."

Alcohol is alcohol.

There is a shot of alcohol in each of these servings, although it is true that if you drink large quantities of beer then you're consuming lots of extra fluid. If you are heavy on the salt intake (which beer drinkers usually are) then you potentially retain more fluid, which, of course, leads to further weight increase.

Note: If you are on a weight-loss plan, nil alcohol is a great idea, because each shot of alcohol carries with it a generous serving of calories - around 70. Maybe once a week, two glasses of wine could be a pleasant bonus.

Note: I am not telling you to drink alcoholic beverages. This is a personal choice. The foregoing merely highlights some of the potential negative and positive effects of alcohol on the human system.

AFDs

AFDs are very clever things. An AFD is an alcohol-free day and these require a touch of discipline.

Many people drink every day of their lives and use alcohol as a crutch. Their tolerance for alcohol increases and as time goes by, they need more and more and more to have the same effect. If you are prepared to throw in an AFD, say one or two a week, it *is a* great discipline.

People say they don't want discipline in their lives, but we actually love discipline and are rewarded by it. When business gets a little tough, people need to get tough. They sharpen their pencils, they make hard decisions, tough decisions. This is successful business management. But self-management? People in business are awful at managing themselves until they are faced with a life-threatening event; then they get very clever at it.

An AFD is a great discipline for everyday drinkers - say a couple of days a week - your body loves you for it. Put two AFDs together and you can almost hear your liver applauding - a sensational feeling. Thank you very much says your body. You usually sleep better as well.

So let's say you have two AFDs, then males may have up to 20-25 drinks to spread out across the rest of the week (females less). That's three or four drinks a day which is pretty fair and reasonable. If you have 10 in one night, then you have to look at the balance over a week and, besides, you feel lousy the next morning. If you have 15 or 20 drinks in one session it literally can kill through acute liver failure. Dean Martin said he felt sorry for non-drinkers because when they wake up in the morning, that's the best they are going to feel all day. But, remember, Dean Martin is dead.

Here's a good party trick. If you are in a social situation and waiters and waitresses are wandering about constantly topping up your glass, don't let them do that, but rather wait until your glass is empty and have it refilled. This way you're in control, and every Sunday you can sit down and count up how many drinks you had last week. Some people frighten the hell out of themselves if they're honest with the counting.

I say to them, "Well, let's look at last week", and we count and we count and we move up to about 35 and they say, "Yeah but that was a bad week." I say, "OK, let's look at the week before", and we count up to about 40 or 50. "But that was a bad week too", they say.

I told you people kid themselves and it's also one hell of a lot of calories, because in one shot of alcohol there are about 70 calories. If you drink 50 drinks a week, that's 3500 calories extra for that week and did you know that there are 3500 calories in one pound of fat? (that's half a kilogram).

So if you drink 50 drinks a week for a year, that's 52 pounds of extra fat you've put on that you have to burn up just to stay level! That's tough, really tough.

In summary, alcohol is not such a bad drug if used very cleverly and if you are in total control. Use the AFDs; count your drinks; socialise; stay in control.

THE BACK END
OF AN AUTOMOBILE

T obacco and nicotine are simply disasters.

Do you know the worst thing about smoking cigarettes? It's the muck that comes out the back end, the end you put in your face. And it's basically the same muck that comes out the back end of an automobile, including that deadly gas carbon monoxide, as well as the lethal chemical, hydrogen cyanide.

These are deadly poisons and yet people continue to do it to themselves. If you are that intent on filling yourself up with these sorts of things, consider those who get a length of tube and stick it on the exhaust pipe, up through the window of the car, then wind the window up and turn the ignition on. The carbon monoxide will fill the lungs, travel into the blood system, and kill you in about 15 minutes. It's called suicide.

If you stayed in the same car and wound up the window and just smoked cigarettes one after the other, the carbon monoxide would kill you in a few weeks or months. But people get out of the car, they only smoke 20 a day, and they survive for years. But 250,000 cigarettes later and something goes horribly wrong - what's the point?

Of course, there is one good thing about smoking a cigarette. It's the deep breath you take after you light up. That first drag and the big inhale.

Deep breaths are fantastic. Do you know what deep breathing does for you? If you take two long, deep breaths, your pulse rate slows down and your blood pressure drops. As well, the spasm begins to disappear from your body and the blood flow is more even.

Cigarette smokers begin to get this effect from the deep breath and for 20 seconds or so everything is slowing down beautifully and then 20 or 25 seconds later when the nicotine hits the blood stream - ZAP. Back to normal?

No way, not back to normal, but way above normal. So if you are a chronic cigarette smoker, your pulse rate at rest is usually too high and so is your blood pressure. It takes a long time - an hour or more - for everything to come back to normal. If you are smoking a cigarette or two every hour, you are probably living life with a pulse rate and blood pressure already elevated. You're living life up there ... and you're starting from up there.

In other words, your baseline is too high, which means you run out of energy and you get tired more quickly. It's just rolling everything up.

It's a disaster. I've said it before and I'll say it again: cigarette smoking is the greatest expression of non-coping there is.

If you must have something stuck in your mouth in order to take a deep breath, instead of a cigarette try your thumb, but that looks stupid doesn't it?

I honestly think that in two or three years, people walking along the street with a cigarette hanging out their mouth will look stupid. In fact, it looks stupid now, especially young kids with cigarettes hanging out of their mouths. Beautiful youth with lungs full of shit. I can't say that? Well I just did and it's a fact.

I'll give you a tip. If your lungs were hanging on the outside instead of the inside and you could actually see what cigarettes were doing to you, no one would smoke.

SUGAR IN THE MORNING, SUGAR IN THE EVENING, SUGAR AT SUPPERTIME

S ugar is good. It is a stimulant. It gets you going and it is used for producing energy. If you have lots of the simple sugars - the sweets, the candies, the cookies and cakes, the soft drinks, the pastries - the sugar is rapidly absorbed into your blood stream and it's there. It's ready; it's energy.

What happens if you don't burn the energy up within a few hours? What does the body do with the energy?

It stores it up in energy stores, and how does the body store most of its energy? As fat, of course. If you have three or four years energy stored up and hanging around your stomach and hips, that's not so good. You might think there's a siege coming, but there probably isn't.

I'll tell you something interesting. You might notice how all the smart people in the world, including the great athletes, the great tennis players (the trend was actually started by the tennis players, the Navratilovas, the Lendls), the great footballers and now even the great business people, are swinging their sugar intake (let's call sugars and carbohydrates the same thing, which they basically are) more towards the multi-molecular complex carbohydrates or sugars - the rice, the vegetables, the grains, the pastas. These are absorbed more slowly into the blood stream at an average of around 2 calories every minute. The rate of absorption has to do with the glycaemic index, but that's too hard to explain. Basically, the more refined the carbohydrate, the faster the energy moves into the system. For example, refined pasta or white bread goes in faster than vegetables.

Two calories a minute is about the amount of energy you burn sitting on your backside. Energy in = energy out.

That's why it's very hard to find a fat vegetarian, because most of their sugar intake is in complex form which takes longer to absorb.

Go for some simple sugars if you want and especially if you're terribly active. But a balance is smart, isn't it? I mean, look at the simple sugar consumption in the United States of America. For a start, each person in the USA averages an intake each day of two or more cans of soda pop, soft drink, lolly water, whatever you call it. That's over half a billion cans of liquid sugar a day consumed in the USA and people wonder why they get fat?

There is so much energy in a can of soft drink - up to 200 calories - which is just fine if you burn it up straight away. So sugar is sugar, it's energy, either a constant supply from complex sugars or giant bursts from simple sugars. Because you mainly sit in cars, sit in planes, and sit behind desks, where does it end up?

And beware, once it is turned into fat it is harder to burn and that's a fact, because the body uses mostly the available sugars and carbohydrates first and then only starts into the fat later on.

We were talking about warning signs, remember? I almost forgot, because of all the other things that interrupted us.

The first two warning signs were MUSCLE SPASM and the CATS Syndrome.

Now for the third warning. ***THE SKIN SIGNS.***

So many adult itches and rashes are precipitated (brought to the surface) by not coping. You may have an underlying genetic predisposition to a skin problem but the condition can flare up when you're under extreme, long-term pressure. It's a warning sign. Skin specialists have a lot of fun - nobody dies from an itch and there are no after-hours calls. They give out nice pills and lotions which do good things, but if you take a holiday and unwind, there is often a similar effect, not for all skin diseases but for the tension sorts of problems. People tell me they have an allergy - a lot of things aren't allergies, but rather they can be tension related.

What about No. 4? ***TIME URGENCY.*** Look at all the people in the world who have too much to do and not enough time to do it every day of the week. You might have too much to do in five or six days maybe, or perhaps you have an important project that takes 15 days in a row. That's fine, but unless you take your 'B' time, your out-of-the-pressure-cooker time, this means you are time urgent all the time and that's a *big warning*.

HOSTILITY. *The hostility warning is No. 5.* I've already told you that a giant difference between Type A maniacs who survive and Type A maniacs who don't is the hostility streak.

You'll notice Type A people whose pack of cards come tumbling down around them are the ones who begin to turn hostile. Things irritate them all the time, big things and little things like creaky desks, flies, noise, lights, air conditioners, papers, people, kids. A great measure of

your tolerance is a noise level which is generally constant. For examp
you walk into your home. There are three kids there making a noise
and they make the same noise day in, day out. But your tolerance
changes. Sometimes you can stand it, sometimes you cannot stand it.
You've changed, they haven't.

If you find that you're increasingly irritated in these circumstances, then
it's time to jump out of your pressure cooker.

You can get aggressive, you're allowed to get aggressive if your aggression
is just for a short time, but if you constantly become aggressive and it
goes on and on, you are gone, you'll start to crumble as so many people
do - the hostile, aggressive Type As.

Don't stew over things for too long. Go take a walk or ride a bike, have
a massage, a glass of wine, turn on a comedy on TV or all of the above.

Warning No. 6 is **CYNICISM**. What a warning! The normal person
turned cynic. Usually OK, but now ... it'll never work ... we've tried it
before ... it's hopeless ... that sort of thing. *Big warning*.

FANATICS DIE YOUNG

I've been around the world many times and met lots of people. I've chatted and observed and interviewed hundreds of those who have made it into their 80s and 90s, and do you know what? ... I believe that people who live long lives and good lives are moderate people - some of this, some of that, and a little of something else.

And another thing...

I can't find any old fanatics. I guess there are a few out there somewhere but I suspect most fanatics are already dead, or else they've given up their fanatical ways.

So I've basically come to the conclusion that if you're over about 35 to 40 years of age, you don't really need to be fanatical about anything.

Sure, you can (and must) have your goals and ambitions and you can be passionate about various aspects of your life, but mix it up.

You know the "all work and no play makes Jack a dull boy" routine ... never a truer word was spoken. The luckiest people are those who consider their job fun.

Fanatics, of course, often become socially unacceptable - fanatical exercisers, fanatical eaters, religious fanatics and the like.

Let's focus on chronic marathon runners (they're people who run more than one marathon).

If you are over 35 and run lots of marathons, hopefully your body can cope with it, because if it can't, then that's a problem.

Have you ever been out to dinner with a chronic marathoner?

Often they fall asleep about 8.30 pm after they've told you about their bad back, their shin splints and their best times. I don't promote fanaticism, although some people seem to be able to deal with it OK.

The problem is that many people over 35 who are fanatical exercisers can break down tissues in the tendons and muscles and joints faster than the regeneration process. And what's the point in that? As a medical doctor, I've certainly seen more broken down old over-exercisers than moderate exercisers.

Have I told you about my lifetime achievement ambitions? I only have three and I've already achieved two of them - and one was to never run a marathon. Another was to win the Melbourne Cup, the most famous and richest handicap horse race in the world. The great Doriemus did it for us in 1995 and he almost won the cup again two years later when he was beaten by a bee's dick (and that's not a big margin) by a horse named Might and Power. I won't tell you my third ambition.

I find there are certain threads which have run through the lives of many of the mature-age people with whom I've had discussions.

Here are the common habits of many long-living people:

1.   They are not aggressive - some tell you they used to be but they've calmed down a long time ago.

2.   They have always eaten fairly simple foods and rarely fast foods. I guess there were no fast foods to eat in those days. Fish and chips now and then was about it.

3.   Very few vegetarians among them, but as a rule the long lifers have always eaten their 'vegies' - and lots of them. Of course, there are religious groups around who are vegetarian and definitely have their share of oldies.

It is interesting that many young people these days, especially girls, give up eating red meat altogether, and I have no idea why they do that. Man, as a hunter, has always eaten red meat since *Day One*. Well, *Day Two* anyway - I think there was an apple involved on *Day One*.

And by the way, the iron in red meat is readily available - it jumps straight into your blood stream - compared to the iron in some other foods, which is more difficult to extract.

If you don't eat any red meat you have to be very careful, because anaemia can creep up on you, causing tiredness and depression, and lack of complete protein can cause all sorts of problems.

4.   They have eaten breakfast most days of their lives.

5.   They have always been fairly active, these days mainly walking and gardening.

6.   There are not too many fat people in Western countries on top of the ground in their 80s (about nil) - they are mainly under the ground.

7.   No alcoholics and not many teetotallers either.

8.   Genetics is a help but not necessarily as big a help as it used to be. You can do OK even if your parents didn't live to a ripe

old age. This is because of the increasing awareness of the control we have over our own risk factors. Example: If your parents died of bowel cancer, you do not need to die from bowel cancer. You have a regular colonoscopy once you hit 40-45 years of age.

9. They usually have routine in their lives - nothing too far out of the ordinary (for them).

10. Those with *meaning* in their lives have a rapport or a bond with others, maybe a loved one, relatives, children or perhaps a pet and they have interests like watching sports (racing, football, cricket, golf) gardening and the like. In fact, it seems if you have nothing to live for, you don't.

Life is crazy at times, isn't it?

I was booked into what is often billed as the best hotel in Australia, overlooking Sydney Harbour. The concierge showed me to my room, and as I was about to pull the curtains back to check the view, I was handed the *curtain remote control.*

That's right, the CRC - the curtain remote control!

You weren't allowed to use your muscles to move the curtains, you had to push a button. Unbelievable! No wonder we get old fast.

And, of course, the new first-class and business-class seats on many airlines actually mould us into the useless sedentary shape we're becoming. You are not allowed to sit up straight unless you're in economy or coach.

The other day I was reading a recent book by Dr Kenneth Cooper, the American guru who 'invented' the word aerobics. In his book,

Antioxidant Revolution, Dr Cooper has done a back flip - I couldn't believe it. He is actually telling people to slow down and not be fanatical about exercise. For years, Dr Cooper has been an advocate of *the more the better* - push, push, count up those points, keep on keeping on.

The good news is Dr Cooper started America running — the bad news is it ran too far and too hard.

I met the man in the late '70s at the Aerobics Institute in Dallas, Texas - sat in his office and listened to his story. Impressive, but I guess I just didn't go for the excesses that Cooper suggested.

Dr Cooper is now telling us that excessive exercise may lead to a weakening of the immune system and a higher risk of cancer at an earlier age.

He has noticed a rise in viral illness in those preparing to run a marathon - in the weeks preceding the race when the training is most intense, and even more so in the *week following* the race.

Does intensive exercise on a chronic basis weaken the immune system? — I say yes!

And while Dr Cooper's book tells us we can be moderate about our exercise now, of course we still have to be OBSESSIVE and play the numbers game by counting our aerobic points.

Some examples in his book:

- Walk 1 mile in between 12.01 minutes and 12.45 minutes - you score 4.25 points.
- Walk 2.5 miles in less than 35.35 minutes twice a week - you score 16.8 points.

- Swim 500 yards in less than 12.30 minutes four times a week - you score 16.7 points.

I've got a headache just reading this stuff! Can't I just go for a brisk walk, or jog for a while, be lightly puffing and feel good and not have to score any points? Give me a break. I spend the rest of my life adding up stuff.

Nowhere in Dr Cooper's book can I find anything about laughing or hugging or doing something nice for someone else.

How many points can I score in the game of life if I hug my kids five days a week for 10.7 seconds?

Maybe while we're scoring so many points, we are actually missing the point.

MANAGEMENT SKILLS

Why are we reading this book? To improve our management skills. You may well say, "But I'm not a manager".

Of course, you are a manager. Everyone manages themself and even co-existence with others demands management skills. You manage people, you manage families, you manage a group, you manage a company.

SELF-MANAGEMENT is what we're talking about right here because that's where management starts, right back with yourself.

One of the things that my rapport with 20,000 or so executives has shown me is that when people move into the Dangerous Decade and lose their ability to self-manage, everything else goes wrong too.

And the pressure is on earlier these days. Look at industries like the money market where it's difficult to survive past about 40 years of age.

It is so easy to shrivel up and become ineffective. It's the pressure, the cigarettes, the coffee, the constant pressure of the money markets where 'seamless' trading now goes 25 hours a day. They used to have a break but not now; the rollercoaster dollars and yen and futures and bond rates and exchange rates go up and down and around and around.

So people don't last - their bodies can't stand the pressure and they can't manage themselves. They don't heed warning signs, and the Dangerous Decade is becoming a younger decade. It used to be the 50s, now it's the 40s, and we're having heart attacks in our 30s. It's a joke.

So what are the skills that we need to survive?

There are only three.

Activity Skills, Eating Skills and Coping Skills - how to bounce around inside the pressure cooker, and more importantly, how to escape.

Activity is something we have removed from our lives. We used to ride bikes to work; we used to go to the corner store on foot to get the milk and bread; we used to chop wood for the fire; we used to walk up stairs - but rarely these days.

You have three choices with activity. You can do nil which is called being a 'slob'.

You can become a fanatic, and as I mentioned before, if you are over the age of 35 to 40, I think fanaticism is a doubtful quality. Maybe your body can cope, but for what? Is it a gold cup? A big medal? Is it applause?

If there is something there you are after and you are a fanatic (even though you are over 35), then go for it if your body can cope, but remember that many bodies can't and they break down. All the tissues, the tendons, the muscles and joints just break down and that breakdown process is usually far quicker than the process of rejuvenation when you move past 40.

Is that fair to your body, or is it just another pressure you're throwing at it?

So slobbery is no good and fanaticism is doubtful. How about the stuff in the middle?

MODERATION

I'll put a number to it for you. Let's make it a minimum of one per cent of your time, a commitment to move this thing called your body.

You can't trade in this body like a car or a spouse, not yet anyway, and we only get one each, so what about moving it for one lousy per cent of the time it's alive?

I assure you, it's a bloody good idea.

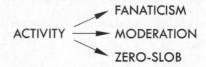

Now, there are 168 hours in a week, every week. I've counted them lots of times and I always get the same. One per cent of 168 hours is 1.68 hours or around 100 minutes each week.

George says, "Hang on, I'm an achiever, I'm successful, I haven't got 100 minutes to move my body. I just haven't got 100 minutes to exercise, I'm too busy."

Well you're a rotten manager.

The 100 minutes can be broken up into 35 minutes by three if you want. Take a brisk walk for 35 minutes, three times a week.

You can ride a bike for 20-25 minutes, 4 times a week, and remember that to be really good for you, you need to be lightly puffing along the way.

If you are not lightly puffing when you are exercising, it is relatively useless. If you are strolling along looking in the shop windows, it's a lovely day out, but you're not really lubricating joints, you are not flushing arteries, and you are not getting lots of oxygen in your head.

When you move and when you are lightly puffing, you actually have an increased amount of oxygen inside your skull and it makes you think smarter.

Often, people can find a solution to a problem while they are walking, because there is more oxygen upstairs. It is a lovely feeling, I assure you.

You *are* permitted to walk up stairs and most places do not have laws against it, although, in the new big buildings, they lock the fire escape doors so you're not allowed to walk up the stairs.

Why?

Because they think some idiot is going to walk into the fire escape and walk up the stairs into the fire.

Not so. You walk down the stairs in a fire, not up, so why do they lock the doors?

I can't understand it.

Why don't they let us people walk up four or five flights of stairs, because that might take two minutes, and if you did that six times every day at the office, there's your exercise without really trying.

I was in Hong Kong recently and I came across on the ferry to Queen's Wharf with all the Asian people on their way to work. They've built overpasses so the people can get over the busy roadway to their offices.

I guess Western people built the overpasses because they aren't bamboo, they're made of concrete.

There are brilliant wide stairs and they've got these skinny little escalators up the side, and the Asians swarm off the boats and they elbow and shove each other to get on these little escalators because everyone likes going up them.

I stood there for 10 minutes and counted the ratio of people on the escalators to the non-hassled people on the big wide stairs. The ratio was 120 to 1.

The Westernisation of Eastern Culture!

What is wrong with walking up stairs? Nothing, and you don't need to wait for the elevator, or push and shove to get a ride.

Forget the fitness thing; rather, think of activity as opening a pressure valve on the pressure cooker, and flushing arteries and lubricating joints and getting oxygen in your head and feeling good.

Remember you need to be at least lightly puffing.

People say, "Well listen, I walk to the bus station, I walk to the train station", but if you are in a suit coat or full set of clothes - blouse, skirt or whatever - then generally you don't walk fast enough to get lightly puffed, because when you are lightly puffed it means you are also lightly sweating and you don't like to sweat in a full set of clothes because it isn't comfortable. So it really means getting into a pair of shorts or a track suit - *that's* the big deal.

If you are not prepared to commit yourself to some activity then you need a coach, and often the best coach is in the same office building, around the corner, next door.

If two people commit to take a walk at 5.30 in the evening or ride a bike, you're more likely to do it when there's the two of you. If you don't turn up you put $20 in the jar and if they don't turn up they put $20 in the jar, and if you're bad self-managers, you'll have a hell of a Christmas party!

SIMPLY THE BEST

W hat sort of exercise is the best?

There's nothing better than walking. Walking is brilliant exercise. Walking is definitely a contender for the Exercise Gold Medal (EGM).

Way back in time we stood up. We weren't meant to, but we did stand up on two legs and we put pressure on the lower back which means that sometimes running hurts the back.

If your body is capable of running then that's fine, but usually when you are starting out on an exercise program, running is a bad idea. Even with walking, your back is very vulnerable, so go buy a pair of shoes, with good support in the heel, and even though they may cost a fair slice of money, they'll last you for years.

It's a great investment.

One interesting point about backs and jogging versus walking. Once you have built up to a stage where you may wish to break into a jog - if you can jog slowly with more of a shuffling action, no high knee action, and leaning forward, then you can actually take the weight and jarring mainly through the stomach muscles rather than the back.

This can protect your back if you get clever at it, whereas walking can put strain on the back if you're very upright.

Type A people often think walking is too boring because they're not getting anywhere fast, but remember it's not how far you go, but the time taken to exercise.

Another tip about your back.

Never stand around for long periods, because this is really bad news for the back. Stand with one foot on a step or stool - this straightens the lower back a bit. And change feet often.

Or lean against a wall and press your lower back against the wall for a few seconds. This feels good.

When you wear an excellent pair of shoes, they gently tip you forward and you're almost walking anyway.

Riding a bike is fantastic, because it takes the support off the joints, gets your heart ticking and gets your legs toned.

Swimming is great exercise - no joint problems with swimming, unless you are a useless swimmer and arch your back too much. There is, however, a downside to swimming.

You've never seen a fat long distance runner anywhere in the world (there aren't any), but there seem to be quite a few fat long-distance swimmers, especially as they age. Why?

They get too good at it. They become so effective that there is less effort required to go a certain distance, and it's harder to burn calories.

You can swim the English Channel but by design you get bigger and bigger and besides, the fat keeps you warm.

There was one chap who swam back and forth across the English Channel so many times, he couldn't remember which language he spoke. He still got fat and ended up having a heart attack. If you are a brilliant swimmer (it's good for your muscle tone and heart) you have to combine it with some brisk walking or jogging or cycling, but if you are an awful swimmer, that's fine; you don't need anything else.

Aerobics is no problem - about 25 to 35 minutes of nice exercise (that step thing included), of mild to moderate intensity. But the people who do an hour or an hour and a quarter of intense pounding, pounding their back into the dust, their shins into the dust - they don't last a long time before injuries set in.

Let's talk about the pulse. You know what the pulse rate is: same as the heart rate. That's the number of times in a minute your heart beats.

If you want to take your pulse rate, you take your pulse at the wrist or one side of the neck, or temple. Perhaps the easiest place is just above the wrist joint between the bone on the thumb side and the tendons. Pop two fingers there and count. Take your pulse for 10 seconds and multiply by six - that gives you the pulse per minute.

If you are exercising, and if you stop and take your pulse for a whole minute, you'll get a false low reading because your pulse is slowing down while you're counting, so just take your pulse for 10 seconds and multiply by 6. It is more accurate.

Now, your maximum pulse rate is the fastest your heart can beat. If you are on a racket ball court or squash court and really going for it and sweating like hell, your maximum pulse is about 220 minus your age.

So if you are 40 years of age your pulse rate at maximum exertion is about 220 minus 40 = 180.

Zero pulse rate is dead, and the resting pulse rate is a good measure of what your base level is and how effective you are (as long as you haven't had a cigarette or coffee in the past hour, and you are reasonably relaxed).

Perhaps the best time to take your resting pulse rate is when you get up in the morning and sit at the breakfast table. Not as soon as you jump out of bed because you may have been dreaming, and your pulse is a little higher.

Sit at the breakfast table, take your pulse for 10 seconds and multiply by six.

The resting pulse rate in an effective person is generally somewhere between 55 and 75. 60 is better than 70.

Women have pulse rates a little higher than men because their hearts are smaller, and they carry more body fat (which makes women pleasantly different), so there is a difference here of maybe 10 beats per minute.

Some top athletes have a resting pulse rate in the high 20s and 30s which is almost dead, but I think that's too low because you have to work out too hard to get lightly puffing.

Now let's say you're a slob, or a heavy coffee drinker, or a chronic smoker, or all of these, then your pulse rate at rest will probably be 20 or 30 beats higher each minute just to start with.

So what's the problem?

I'll tell you what the problem is. That's 10 to 15 million beats a year that your heart is overworking and besides, you're coming from higher rather than lower and you run out of energy quicker - it's a fact.

You get tired maybe even before lunch.

I said that to be effective, you should be at least lightly puffing when you are active. The pulse rate when you are lightly puffing is around 70% of maximum. So if your maximum pulse rate is potentially 180 (40 years of age) or 170 (50 years of age) then the pulse rate or heart rate when you are lightly puffing needs to be only 120-130.

The best thing about being a slob is that to get lightly puffing, all you have to do is get out of your chair and your heart gets such a fright, it goes straight to 130, because it's almost there to start with.

Way back, I did a treadmill test on a man in one of my Risk Evaluation Clinics in Australia.

George says, "Hang on - I wouldn't want the treadmill test - it sounds scary!"

Well if you want to improve your system, you can't unless you've got some baseline data.

You have to know where you are coming from to measure where you are going to, irrespective of whether it is a business, office, computer or personal system that you wish to improve. One of the best ways to collect data about the effectiveness of an individual body (and it doesn't matter whether you're fit or unfit) is to put that body on a treadmill, hook it up to a pulse rate monitor, cardiograph machine and oxygen consumption monitor, and make the body walk.

Treadmill testing usually takes somewhere between four and 14 minutes. If you are a slob, the treadmill test is relatively easy because your heart rate rises quickly and after you walk for four minutes you are probably at maximum.

If you are a fanatical exerciser or a marathon runner, we may have to run you up an incline for 10, 12, 14 minutes and because your heart is strong it takes a while to get there.

It is a good test because you can accumulate baseline data which is motivating in itself; you can monitor improvements over a period of time, and compare yourself with yourself, rather than with other people and with pictures on billboards.

We really should forget how old we are because chronological age means little. It is physiological or 'real age' which is the measuring stick and the human body is such an amazing thing. Seventy year olds can do the same things as 40 year olds if they do it often enough. That's called the training effect.

I have seen people dramatically reverse the ticking clock of 'real age' *after* they have had their coronary (heart attack) simply because there is an incentive and a reason to do so.

They exercise, they eat well, they crank up the mind power and while the chronological clock goes on 10 years, their physiological clock goes backwards 20. It's great stuff.

A woman in her 80s riddled with arthritis complained to me that her doctor didn't ever tell her to exercise until she turned 80. The water exercises freed up her joints so well.

"Why didn't he tell me when I was 60?"

Back to the treadmill test. I did a test on this character in Australia, obese man, 47 years of age, computer expert, stressed to the eyeballs, 60 cigarettes a day. He walked into my clinic on his way to lunch - his company had sent him as part of the tax-effective program they run for their people.

It is interesting that most individuals really aren't motivated to spend this type of money, but companies will spend it.

Twenty years ago companies weren't people - companies were machines. If you gave the boss the choice of getting rid of the people, or the machines, plant and equipment, he'd get rid of the people because you could replace them next day. Now you can replace the machines tomorrow (they're outdated anyway) but you can't get rid of highly trained people and replace them tomorrow.

Nowadays, companies *are* people.

A little bit of money spent in this area of awareness is very, very valuable.

So I said to this chap, "Give me your questionnaire please." And he said, "No way, I'm not going to fill out any forms."

"Would you do the treadmill test?" He said, "OK" and he put on his brand new track shoes that he'd bought on the way to the test - sparkling new, coloured stripes, never been used before. I showed him on to the treadmill and connected him to the computer monitors and cardiograph machine.

Now this man was standing still, he wasn't moving yet, and already his pulse rate was 118 - unbelievable! - 118 beats every minute just to keep him alive!

I was concerned about this man. I knew from my data that the minimum treadmill test time was around four minutes but I was careful and I walked him on the treadmill quite slowly without any incline.

In just one minute and 10 seconds his pulse rate went over 200! I stopped the test. He said, "Why are you stopping the test?" I said, "Because you might drop dead." He said, "Bloody good decision."

He had absolutely no idea. His whole system was so ineffective that if you applied some slight physical pressure, some mental pressure ... whoosh ... his heart rate was flying.

Why did this guy get tired every day before lunch? Why did he go out to lunch five days a week? Why did he have a bottle of wine at lunch to rev himself up and get a bit of fool's energy - squeeze that little bit of energy out of those grapes for the next hour before he drifted into a half sleep or went home? I mean this guy was totally ineffective.

The other great thing about this test was that the man's electrocardiograph (ECG) tracing was perfectly normal at rest, absolutely perfect, but 60 seconds into his test he had a nasty cardiograph tracing. I knew he had heart disease but he didn't know, because he had never noticed any symptoms.

Did you know that the first symptom or sign in up to 30% of people with heart disease is sudden death? It's awfully hard to cure. Two thirds of people get a warning ... the other third do not ... they just put the cue in the rack and lie down.

This guy with the lousy treadmill test could easily have had a heart attack changing a tyre on his car, or rushing to catch a bus, because he wasn't aware, he didn't care.

You know, there was this colleague who did static health testing on executives and a few years back an executive walked into his office for a check-up. The doc tapped his chest - normal; took the blood pressure - normal; cholesterol - normal; and then laid him on the bench and did a resting electrocardiograph - normal. The guy got up, put on his clothes, walked outside and dropped dead!

I said, "My God! What did you do?"

He said, "Oh ... we turned him around so he looked like he was coming in."

In the heart disease stakes, it is interesting that women are protected to an extent by the female hormones, but of course men aren't. Men can take female hormones if they want, but if they do then the wrong things grow and the right things shrivel up.

The ratio of heart attacks in males to females in the under 50 age group is about 10 to one. In the post menopausal age group the statistics show that the number of women having heart attacks moves up to about level with men.

If you have symptoms relative to the heart, maybe chest pains, tightness, palpitations, light headedness, whatever - if you go to the doctor and the doctor lies you on a bench and does a resting electrocardiograph and says your heart is perfect, then I must admit that I wouldn't accept that as gospel. I would rather my heart were tested under pressure on a treadmill, because you have a lot more information with a heart under pressure.

Back to this guy with the bad ECG under pressure. I thought he was in trouble, so we decided to do an angiogram. An angiogram is where you put dye into the blood system, the heart fills up with dye, we take pictures, you see the heart, and you see the coronary arteries.

You've heard people say, "A coronary, he had a coronary." That means a heart attack. The coronary arteries are in and around the heart and do you know how big these arteries are? The three biggest arteries in your heart, the arteries that supply your heart with blood and life, are about one fifth the width of your little finger. Not very big at all.

So a coronary is the same as a heart attack and happens when the arteries become blocked.

The angiogram showed that this chap had virtually a 100% blockage in his right coronary artery, a 90% blockage in the middle one and around 60% blockage in the other one. He was living on four tenths of one artery, and a trickle through another, but didn't know it.

The sludge gradually builds up over a period of time and people say, "Yeah, well it's genetics for a start, and besides it doesn't happen until you're 40." I tend to disagree ... the sludge seems to start when you are a teenager or even younger - especially in Western countries, depending on what your parents fed you to make you fat and happy.

Most males over 15 have a degree of artery blockage. As life goes on, if you have less than a 50% blockage then it doesn't matter too much, but if you have over 50% blockage, it's getting to be more of a worry.

Very few pre-menopausal women have significant heart disease. That's a big statement, but it's basically correct, an exception being the smokers. You see the oestrogen hormones, the female hormones pushed out by the ovaries, are very protective of arteries. They tend to keep women's arteries clean while their ovaries are working, but nicotine tends to offset that oestrogen effect, so if you are a woman you'd be absolutely crazy to smoke, wouldn't you?

If you were a man you'd be even more crazy to smoke because you haven't got any protective oestrogens in the first place.

That treadmill guy was lucky. He had localised blockages and was a good candidate for a bypass operation. If the coronary arteries are stuffed up all the way along, then there's nothing to bypass.

So he had the operation, ate some decent food, cut back on the booze, walked around the neighbourhood most days, lost a lot of excess baggage, changed his job, re-introduced himself to his family and learnt his kids' names all over again.

The reason he changed jobs (apart from the chronic pressure he couldn't handle), he was spending so much time travelling, every time he arrived back home the dog bit him.

Now this man is really living again.

If you build up that sludge to a stage where there is an 85 to 90% blockage and you don't know it, then all you need is one clot of blood to come floating down that little old artery and go clunk, and the lights are out - especially if your other two arteries aren't in shape as well.

Blockages? What can you do about them? Well, you can have a bypass, a coronary bypass if the conditions are favourable.

Do you know what a bypass is? That's where the surgeons take a blood vessel from somewhere else in your body, and sew it onto your coronary artery and actually bypass the blockage. But as I just mentioned, what if the blockage isn't localised? What if the whole artery is shot to bits? There's nothing much you can do is there? George is now saying to me, "Well what do you want me to do? It's genetics mate, it's genetics." Sure it's genetics, but how much, a half, a third?

What about the other control bit? What about the stuff you put in your face? What about food??

FOOD GLORIOUS FOOD

The skill of *eating is* the second of the survival skills (self management skills) we need. There are two food groups in the world.

Some nutritionists say there are four food groups and others say there are five food groups, but I say there are two food groups and I am right because I've been in marketing and I know about the KISS philosophy (Keep It Simple Stupid).

Way back when I played professional football in Australia (Aussie Rules - now there's a *real* game of football - no padding or protective whatever, just muscles and bones and flesh crunching together) my coach used to say that when you're under extreme pressure you can only remember a maximum of two things at once if you're smart, and a maximum of one thing at once if you're not so smart. He used to be grateful if the players on his team turned up at the correct stadium.

So back to food groups - there are two, OK?

Before I tell you about food groups, a word about diets.

DIETS

Did you know people spend millions and millions of dollars every day buying diet books, and of course all the diet books say something different. One says this, another says that, and the authors can get quite wealthy. Now, who invented the word DIET?

I don't know who did, but if we could find them, him, her, we should banish them forever, because diet is a terrible word. If you go on a diet, you go off the diet.

When you go on a diet, you want some action, you want to lose weight as fast as you can, and when you lose weight fast, what do you lose? You lose fluid, you lose fat and you lose muscle as well, and the faster the weight comes off, the more muscle bulk you lose. Then you put the weight back on within a few weeks or months, and when you put the weight back on, what do you put back on? First you put back the fluid, then you put back the fat, but you don't put back as much muscle, especially if you are a fast weight loser.

When you are back to square one, your percentage of body fat is actually higher then when you started. CRAZY! So, what's the answer?

The answer is a change of attitude and that's why we look at this very simply, because you don't want to be confused while you are changing your attitude.

I repeat, there are *two* food groups in the world.

One food group is called BASIC and the other food group is called BONUS.

Basic foods are plant foods - vegetables, fruits, grains, grain breads, pastas, rice. If you live on these to the exclusion of all else, then you are a fanatic. You tend to run out of friends, you never get invites out to dinner, you are in danger of becoming a social outcast.

Ever heard of Nathan Pritikin? I admired the man. I met Nathan Pritikin on several occasions and I thought he was brilliant. He literally turned American nutrition on its ear, sensational stuff. He had artery disease and he decided to do something about it personally, so he invented the Pritikin Regression Diet. To eat that way and stick to it, you've got to be unwell or a touch crazy because it really is tough.

I've done a lot of research into Pritikin. I know now if you eat Pritikin long enough, you can't get cancer ... you just look like you've got it.

That's why the great thing about my program is that I really don't care what you eat. You can actually eat anything you like, you can even eat bonus foods.

What's a bonus food? A bonus food is everything that is not a basic food, which makes it very easy to work out. Red meat, cheese, ice cream, chocolates, cream cakes, etc. etc. Great aren't they?

I don't care if you eat them; the critical thing is BALANCE.

Where is the balance? Where is the pendulum?

If you are a Western-style eater, your pendulum is most likely way over there on the bonus side.

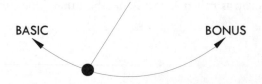

George (almost in tears), "But red meat — isn't it good for you?"

Of course it is. It has protein, high-quality protein; it has iron; it has vitamin B12 which is hard to get in other foods; it is very good for you, so why don't you have some every now and again? Maybe once a week or maybe twice a week or maybe three serves a week, but you wouldn't go past three times a week if you were half smart.

George says, "Yeah, well my gran pappy down on the farm he had bacon and eggs for breakfast, he had sausages for lunch and steak for dinner and more meat for supper. That's three or four times a day he ate red meat and he died when he was 99. So what about that?"

George, I guarantee one thing about your gran pappy - he was physically working 14 hours a day and you don't. It's very hard to get away with that sort of eating if you just sit on your butt. And, besides, the exception doesn't prove the general rule.

What about big pieces of fatty cheese full of saturated animal fat that sticks to the insides of your arteries - you can eat them? Sure, why not? One, two, three times a week, but you wouldn't go past that would you? You wouldn't eat cheese every day just because you are hungry, would you?

Chocolates? Three a week, that's OK. Where is the pendulum?

Remember, basic is plant and bonus is not plant.

THE GREATEST RULE OF NUTRITION

T he greatest rule of nutrition ever invented is this (and I invented it). It's the two-thirds, one-third rule (2/3,1/3).

THE TWO-THIRDS, ONE-THIRD RULE

If you are prepared to eat two thirds of the food that you put in your face as plant food, and if you are prepared to eat only one-third or less as flesh food or refined food, then that's all you need to know.

You can virtually forget all the other stuff you've heard about fat and cholesterol, if you want to, because there is no cholesterol (nil, nought, zero) in any plant food and very little fat in plant food, except in olives and avocados. We'll talk about that later.

Maybe you will go into a hotel or restaurant tonight and tell the waiter that Dr John said you can have a bonus, so you order steak.

"A steak please, medium rare, nice and juicy."

So here comes the plate and here's the steak and here are the peas, the asparagus and maybe some potato. You see the restaurant stuffed up the rule, didn't they? They gave you 2/3 plus *plus* flesh, and 1/3 minus *minus* plant, and lots of people leave the plant anyway.

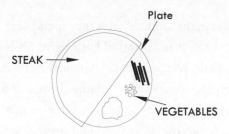

Look at the smorgasbord lunches. The meats and cheeses always go first because people were brought up that way.

What about the Eastern Culture?

Here's the plate, here's all the rice, here are the vegetables all over the place. Then they have small portions of meat, fish, chicken. They've got the rule right - 2/3 plant, 1/3 flesh.

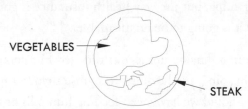

"Now just wait a minute, how come we are living till 80, 85 years of age at this stage if we eat all this crappy food?"

I'll tell you how come.

First, we dramatically reduced childbirth deaths - you don't die having babies nowadays - and then we got rid of infectious diseases - the typhoid, the cholera - and nobody tends to die now of tuberculosis or polio in Western countries. So that moved us back to three score year and ten, and then we added another eight or 10. How did we add the eight? Medical technology - absolutely brilliant medical technology - unaffordable, but brilliant.

Do you know that in the United States they spend over $3 billion a day on health care? (I call it sick care). That's right: $3 billion every day. Remember the Gulf War way back? General Schwarzkopf was at a barbecue at my place (there's some name dropping for you) and he mentioned that the USA spent $3 billion a day on that war and people said, "Gee whiz, I wish the war would end because we can't afford the $3 billion a day, it's breaking us." Now they're spending almost that on sick care.

I'll give you another outstanding fact. Do you know that up to half of that money is spent on people in the very last year or so of their life? Half the money goes on keeping people alive for the last few months of their life and they're going to die anyway. I know it might be your grandma or grandpa, but the way health insurance is going, in five to 10 years' time it is going to be unaffordable.

My uncle was in a nursing home and they fed him lots of pills every day to keep him going, and he didn't recognise anyone any more. What do you think? Should we have been feeding him pills or not?

There will be very few people indeed who will be able to afford health insurance because health care (sick care) costs are galloping way ahead of any inflationary or consumer price index.

That's why self-management is making a big comeback. That's why health insurers in America are starting to do deals with companies who look after their people, teaching their people to self manage. One day the government will realise that non-smokers are subsidising the health insurance fees for smokers and charge the smokers more for health insurance, just like the life insurance companies do. It's the only way health insurance is going to survive. We definitely need to help - ourselves.

Anyway, that's enough philosophy for now.

I'm telling you the best way to eat is the 2/3, 1/3 way. Relate that to any meal you like.

Does it fit in with breakfast? What's the 2/3?

Easy, plant foods, grains, some fruit, cereal, toasts - that's the 2/3.

What's the 1/3? The bonus, the flesh, the ham and eggs. Enter George. "I love ham and eggs; I have 21 eggs a week mate." Well, eggs are great food value, but I tend to think they're a bonus food. Why don't you cut down? "I don't want to cut down; I love ham and eggs." OK then, you give me a food; I can mess around with that food and possibly improve it.

Eggs are good food value, especially for kids. They are even producing eggs now with a lot less cholesterol. If you want an egg or two each week, no problem. If you eat 21 a week, do them my way, especially if you have a cholesterol problem.

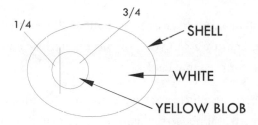

Here is an egg. There's the shell, with lots of calcium if you want to eat it. Then the egg white. Egg white (along with deep sea fish) is the best form of high quality protein known to the human system. It is excellent, all the amino acids, number one protein, fantastic stuff.

The yellow blob in the middle - it has a public relations problem. In my opinion, you can improve an egg. Throw the shell away and prepare the egg with all the white, but with only one quarter of the yolk. It looks pale but tastes much the same. Even with a fried egg, you can pop it on some grain toast, saw off some white and scrape just a little yellow on for the taste.

Why don't you give the three quarters of the yolk to your dog and let him have the heart attack?

Most people wouldn't do that, because they love their dog.

What about a beautiful meal in a restaurant? The chef generally does a superb job and then often covers his masterpiece with gravies and sauces. And of course George says, "But I love the gravy and sauces." So you eat maybe double the calories. Why don't you order the sauce on the side or in little crock pots because you only need an eighth of the sauce for the same taste?

Salads

Don't allow oil or salad dressing to be poured all over the salad. Order it on the side, because again you only need a sixth or an eighth of the oil or dressing for the same taste.

You need to become a little assertive when you walk into a restaurant. You can have two appetisers if you want: a seafood appetiser then perhaps a pasta appetiser.

They say, "Oh, you're not allowed to do that." So you run right through the menu to please the restaurateur. If you choose to, you can order an appetiser and then a plate of vegetables. They usually think you are crazy and they look at you and they point at you and all that.

If they do prepare the vegetable platter and want to impress you and retain your custom, they will do a superb vegetable platter, and at the end of the night, have no idea how much to charge you!

'Vegetable Platter' - usually $8 instead of $15 or $20. You save money and your life as well.

You can be nicely assertive in restaurants. You don't need to be rude, just nicely assertive.

What I want to get through to you is this: the body's desire for food is pretty simple. One of the great differences between chronically overweight people and those that are not....

For the overweight, food generally is *THE MAIN EVENT*

or at least *A* MAIN EVENT, whilst for others, food is what you eat when you are hungry.

Here's something that will help you understand the food and body business.

There are only three systems in the human body that cause you to desire food.

System No.1 is the brain box. It wants food because it receives and translates hunger signals. System No. 2 is the nose and tongue. They work in conjunction. System No. 3 is the stomach. Actually the stomach really does not care what you put in it. As long as it is full two or three times a day, it is happy. You can fill it up with anything - sardines, baked beans, cardboard boxes - just fill it up and it's delighted.

The biggest worry is the front of the tongue which has most of the taste buds on it and tastes sugar and salt and nice fats. So if you have three sugars in your coffee, *you* don't really want all that sugar, you are merely feeding the tip of your tongue. Some people pick up the salt shaker, and they haven't tasted their food yet, and they throw salt all over their meal even though they don't really want the salt. They're feeding the tip of their tongue, because their tongue grew up with salt - it just expects it to be there.

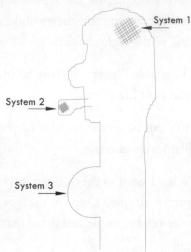

Other people get hold of a box of chocolates and they rip open the box and eat the whole 16 chocolates. They eat them all, even though the stomach gets sick of them after three or four, but they keep eating and eating because once again they are feeding the tip of their tongue.

In most people, the Good Lord built the brain box (the control box) in the superior position way above the tongue. In a lot of people, the tongue is way out of control.

If you love chocolates, good luck to you, but why eat four when two do the trick and why eat five or six when two still do the trick?

Interesting, isn't it?

PS: If you want to win money, ask someone to spell 'restaurateur'. They usually spell it with an 'n'.

FAT

W atch this....

Fat has .... 9 calories per gram

Protein has .... 4 calories per gram

Sugars, carbohydrates have .... 4 calories per gram

Does this mean anything to you? What it means to me is this...

Eat fat, get fat.

Fat keeps you warm and it keeps your internal organs from banging together. It is also an energy store, so the body needs *some* fat.

Fat is obvious in lots of foods but it also hides in many of the processed and packaged foods on supermarket shelves, and there's often heaps of it in fast foods, depending on how they're prepared.

A FAT LOT OF GOOD

The Fats

There are saturated fats, unsaturated fats, and mono-unsaturated fats and in most foods there are combinations of these types of fats. It has something to do with how many carbon and hydrogen bits - how hydrogenated the fat is. Far too complicated for us to understand.

George says to me, "What the hell are you talking about?"

Well, saturated fats are animal fats - they are generally solid at room temperature and body temperature. Here's a great rule for you: *the harder the fat on your plate, the harder it is in your arteries.* You walk along the supermarket aisles, and in some supermarkets, the meats seem to be graded by fat content. Generally speaking, the lower socio-economic groups go straight for the higher fat stuff because it is lower priced. This is a pity.

The fat jumps into your supermarket trolley; you take it home; you cook it and you eat it; and the animal fat wanders around the blood system and lounges in the arteries. And because it is sticky, saturated fat, it can stick to the artery walls. George is at it again: "Are you telling me I can't eat animal fat like in a juicy steak? I love the stuff!"

Listen to me. Man in his natural state was a hunter (this is a non-sexist comment because the man was the hunter). He hunted red meat. He wandered through the plains looking for a buffalo or pig, banged it on the head, and they ate it all at once, because nobody had any money to buy a refrigerator.

Come to think of it, there weren't any refrigerators.

Actually, America started getting the world fatter when it invented refrigerators, so then you could keep fatty food and meats from going off and turning bad and you could also keep drinks full of sugar nice and cool.

America got even fatter when it invented supermarkets because they are very big and they have too many shelves. Most of the shelves started out empty, but the inventors invented lots of crappy, high-calorie foods to fill them up. Eighty per cent of the products on supermarket shelves didn't exist 15 years ago.

America got even fatter when it invented fast foods because most fast-food operators forgot the 2/3 - 1/3 rule and instead went to the 1/20 - 19/20 rule or thereabouts.

Anyway, back to the hunter. The hunters couldn't find buffaloes every day and other red meats every day, so while they were looking, they would live off fruits, the roots of trees, the nuts, the grains, and catch a fish now and then.

You know about carnivores and herbivores.

Well, the human being is omniverous, but actually built more as a herbivorous being, a plant-eating being.

Carnivores, meat eaters, are built differently. Carnivores have a head full of canine teeth. We've only got four. We also have molars and incisors for cutting and chewing plant food. Carnivores, the meat-eating animals, have very short intestines. They grab a lump of meat and rip it to shreds - they don't really chew it too much, they just swallow it - and the part that is digested is digested and the rest goes straight out the back door - whoosh - because they have short intestines.

Human beings have intestines that are very, very long, all folded up around and around inside you. Why? To digest plant food, of course. So if you are eating your red meat now and then that's fine, but if you eat heaps and heaps of the stuff and little else except fully absorbed refined foods, what's it doing? Just hanging around in there.

If you open the intestines of a 55-year-old eating meat 15, 20, 30 times a week, what do you see inside? Lots of flesh, semi-digested, lazily lying against the bowel wall, especially if there is little or no plant fibre (and no exercise) to stimulate the intestines and help all that muck on its way.

We wonder why bowel cancer is the biggest cancer in Western countries now. It's obvious isn't it? - you've got to get the pendulum in the right place - swing it to the plant side.

So do we need to give up eating meat altogether? I don't think so. We've always enjoyed a little meat. But when refrigeration was invented, Western people started to eat meat *every day.* That's where we went wrong.

Two-thirds plant, one-third flesh and refined foods is the way to go.

What about the other sort of fat? Unsaturated fats. They're oils, liquids, they move, they go, whereas saturated fats are more solid and they stick.

Lots of vegetable oils and most fish oils are unsaturated.

However, there are two examples of vegetable fats or oils which are mainly saturated fats and these two may be quite dangerous because saturated fats tend to raise the body's level of cholesterol production. This is where food-labelling laws in the United States are very good, whereas food-labelling laws in many other countries are very bad because they just put 'vegetable oil' on the label.

If the vegetable oils are palm oil or coconut oil, remember they are the two plant oils that are mainly saturated and they possibly act on the body like animal fats.

It is not absolutely clear, because some studies show palm oil to have a reasonable effect on body chemistry.

What I think is this. In their natural environmental context, palm oils and coconut oils are probably fine, because they're not forced into combination with all the other contrived Western food products.

Most big commercial cake manufacturers and biscuit/cookie manufacturers use palm oil and coconut oil because they're cheaper you see. We should know these things, but we're not told them most of the time.

Some of the breakfast cereals have lots of coconut. They're supposed to be healthy cereals and they put in coconut, which contains mainly saturated fat. I'm sure coconut is OK to eat now and then in its natural fibrous state, but I question whether it needs to be in breakfast cereals. Besides, fat contains lots of calories.

What about mono-unsaturated fat? If you want to get fat and be relatively safe about it, try the Mediterranean way.

Many Mediterranean people eat a lot of mono-unsaturated fats and there seems to be no great danger of heart disease with these types of fats. Remember though, once a fat is artificially solidified, it is partially hydrogenated - ie partially 'stuffed up'.

There is also research that shows if you fill up with lots of polyunsaturates such as safflower oil and sunflower oil, you might increase the risks of various cancers, maybe breast cancer, maybe bowel cancer - apparently something to do with 'free radicals'.

The Mediterranean type of fat seems to be relatively safe - avocados, olives, olive oil, canola oil, and peanut oil are mainly mono-unsaturated fats.

People day, "Well, you shouldn't use butter, you should use polyunsaturated margarine", but if you use just a scraping, who cares?

If you are going to use a big lump of it, polyunsaturated fat in margarine probably is less threatening to the heart than saturated fat in butter, but I would go the mono-unsaturated way. I would spread a little avocado on the toast.

George says, "Hang on, what about the cholesterol in avocado?"

I thought you had gone to sleep George. Let me tell you something.

There is *no cholesterol in any plant food.*

They stick little stickers on avocados saying 'cholesterol free', but there's never been any in there to start with!

There is *no cholesterol in any plant food* - get that straight.

Mind you, the only fruits and vegetables that contain more than a few per cent fat are avocados and olives (they're about 70%) but at least it's relatively safe fat. If you want to get real fat, real safe - go for these things, right? But if you get too fat, your blood pressure goes up, and there aren't too many fat people on top of the ground in Western countries after three score years and 10.

Here's another alternative. Instead of butter or margarine on your bread, how about a little olive oil or perhaps even *nothing*. "Nothing??" Yes, you can taste the bread better.

I'll tell you something else worth knowing. Some of the fast-food chains throw their fries into boiling saturated fat - maybe it's a conspiracy!

What is a fry? A fry is a piece of potato. Potato is a great food because it is a complex carbohydrate - it is absorbed relatively slowly and it provides fantastic energy.

People often go on A DIET and the first things they give up are potatoes and bread.

Potatoes and grain breads are sensational foods, so why give them up when they help you lose weight, especially if you are reasonably active?

But what do people do to the potato? They slice this potato into around 20, 30 or 40 pieces, and the more slices they can get, the more the surface area increases. If you slice a potato into this many chips you increase the surface area hundreds of times, which you can then cover in salt. And, of course, the slices are so thin, as soon as you throw them in the fat to cook, the fat meets straight in the middle. You can actually pick up the fries and wring the fat out of them - yuk! If it's saturated fat (animal fat) they're cooking in, you've got to be kidding. It heads straight into the arteries.

"Hey, you're having a go at fast foods," says George. Well, not really. Fast foods are a great *bonus food* for just now and then.

For example, a burger, if it is high-quality, low-fat meat, with some salad and a bun, is OK now and then. And the fries? Perhaps you can get away with some if they are *very chunky* fries and browned in a little polyunsaturated or mono-unsaturated oil.

If you are going to cook in oil, olive oil is way ahead of the rest. Pure virgin olive oil - from the olives that run the fastest!

The only thing you can do to olive oil to stuff it up is to heat it to temperatures so high that it starts to smoke, or reheat the oil time and again when it can become rancid and nasty.

Other fast foods?

Pizza is fine, if you can come by a base that is less refined and the toppings are low-fat cheese and lots of vegetables, peppers and other plant varieties ... fantastic.

Even the good old 'fish and chips', especially grilled fish and a few big chips, is fine as a bonus food now and again.

All types of fats contain the same calories though. It doesn't matter what sort it is, you still get fat whether it's saturated or not. It's how safely you want to get fat.

THE GOOD OIL

D o you need an oil change? Quite possibly.

Obviously we eat too much fat, but as well as cutting down on all fats, we probably need to change the percentages of the various types of fat I'm talking about. That is, change back to a more 'natural' ratio - less saturated animal fat, more mono unsaturated (Mediterranean) and even less of the polyunsaturated vegetable oils we are using today.

The two most important groups of polyunsaturated fatty acids are the Omega 3 and Omega 6 essential fatty acids - sounds like star wars! Our ancestors used to eat about equal amounts of these, but now we tend to use 20 times Omega 6 compared to Omega 3 because of the vast increase in consumption of vegetable oils such as safflower and sunflower. We need to swing back to the Omega 3 which is found in fish, especially sardines, salmon, mackerel, tuna and oils such as canola, soybean, walnut and flaxseed (linseed).

It is interesting that races of people who eat foods rich in the Omega 3 fatty acids (eg Greenland Eskimos) have a low incidence of heart disease, rheumatoid arthritis, psoriasis and asthma.

One can postulate that because the balance has tipped the wrong way in Westernised countries, these diseases are to the fore. Conversely, less Omega 6 and more Omega 3 should help.

Let's crack open a can of sardines, George.

I'm going to print a table that makes me feel very important. If you don't want to read it, don't bother. If you read it and can't understand it, don't worry, it's no big deal.

A Breakdown of Common Fats & Oils

Fat or Oil	Saturated Fatty Acid	Mono-unsaturated Fatty Acid	Polyunsaturated Fatty Acid
Coconut Oil	86	7	2
Cow's milk fat	62	29	4
Beef dripping	48	42	4
Palm oil	48	38	9
Sheep fat	43	39	8
Chicken fat	33	45	18
Soya bean oil	15	23	58
Olive oil	14	73	9
Corn oil (maize)	13	25	58
Safflower oil	9	13	74
Walnut oil	9	23	63
Linseed oil	9	20	66
Canola oil	6	58	32
Evening Primrose Oil	9	7	80

BIG MUSCLES

Younger people tend to ask the following:

"Well, what about the protein mate? I want big muscles and you need protein for big muscles and strength."

Well, proteins are proteins and they are made up of building blocks. Have you ever heard of amino acids? No, I didn't think so, even though you probably learnt about them in school.

There are 22 or so little building blocks that make up proteins and nine of these blocks are essential. In other words the body can't make them. The body can make most of the building blocks but it can't make nine of them - you actually have to eat those nine.

The great thing about high-quality protein - the meats, the fish, the eggs, the cheese, the milk - is that the whole lot of these nine essential amino acids are all in the one food. They are all there; it is that simple. We call this a complete protein food.

Vegetarians have to be careful. They need to put various building blocks together, because most vegetables only contain two or three or four of these essential amino acids, not the whole nine. So you have to eat that with this and this with that to make sure you're getting all the essential amino acids in the *same meal.*

There is nothing wrong with high-quality protein. As I said, egg white is far and away the best high-quality protein, along with fish. The trouble with a lot of complete protein foods is that they contain a lot of fat as well.

"But what about shell fish? I've heard it contains cholesterol."

It's interesting this cholesterol business. About one quarter of the cholesterol in your blood stream you have eaten. The other three quarters you have manufactured in your liver. How come? Why do you make cholesterol? Well, you make it to help digestion, you make it to help produce sex hormones, and the coating around nerves and things like that.

You definitely need some cholesterol, you can't have nil in your body. The cholesterol produced in your liver is plenty. "Why does the liver produce cholesterol?"

If you eat a lot of saturated fat (animal fat), your liver pours cholesterol into the blood stream to help digestion and metabolism. The more meats, cheeses and fatty fast foods, the more cholesterol is produced, so an excess can build up in your system.

Genetics plays a big part. If you have chosen your folks well, great. If you haven't, you have to try harder.

Several Swedish doctors are convinced that negative stress plays a big part in cholesterol production. This resulted from research on employees under threat of being out of work, and cholesterol rose highest in those who suffered disturbances of sleep.

A lot of medicos probably wouldn't agree with this last one, but they might in 10 years' time. Many doctors still don't agree with stress as a risk factor.

"Stress doesn't give you heart attacks."

Well, stress may not build up the sludge, but if an artery is 85% blocked, what is the final thing that can precipitate the heart attack? Spasm of the artery, muscle spasm, tension.

If you look at an artery end on - look down the artery - you see a little hole with muscle wrapped around it. If the muscle is in spasm you have smaller pipes, but still the same amount of fluid and that same pump. If you clamp the pipes down, what happens? The blood pressure goes up. Simple isn't it?

You go to the doctor and the doctor says, "You have high blood pressure, come back next week." Still high. "Come back again." Still high.

What's the treatment? Pills? Maybe, if the problem is genetic.

What if it's not genetic? What if it is just tension? Why don't you become a B Type now and again and have your blood pressure taken when you are totally relaxed. Perhaps even some biofeedback will help. It can show you how the pulse and blood pressure respond to the relaxation.

Some people don't even relax when they are asleep, because they don't drop down into the really deep sleep. How can you if you're full of sleep pills, awake pills, downer pills, upper pills and sideways pills?

Where was I? Shell fish, that's right.

Shell fish contains some cholesterol, but listen to this.

If you give a vegetarian pure egg yolk or oysters or prawns or something with lots of cholesterol, the cholesterol level in the blood doesn't move much. If you give pure cholesterol to a heavy meat and saturated fat eater, the blood level of cholesterol seems to go up. So it appears to be the *combination* of saturated animal fats and cholesterol that is the problem.

You can get away with shellfish some of the time, and regular fish more of the time, like most of the time.

The worst meats are obviously the luncheon meats and salamis where fat jumps out and almost hits you in the face. And sausages with big lumps of fat - Wow! - it just heads straight for your arteries.

Then you come down to your lean lamb and beef - that's not too bad you know - quite low amounts of saturated fat if you chop the visible fat off. Lots of available iron in red meat as well.

CHICKEN

People say you have to eat more chicken. If you eat chicken with the skin left on, then that fills you with more saturated fat than lamb or beef. Surprise! That's because most of the saturated fat is in the chicken skin.

You know those fast-food nuggets? - well some have embarrassing amounts of chicken skin in them. They get the chicken and fatty skin, squash them together. Hey presto - nuggets!

Chicken breast with the skin ripped off (before cooking) has a lower saturated fat content than red meat.

Lower still - fish; lowest - egg white.

So there's the spectrum of complete protein foods from high fat to low fat.

CALORIE BURNING

We've got George thinking.

"I know the three things - the activity, the eating and the coping - but I just love eating and I still want to lose weight."

If you want to lose weight and still eat, then slam the pendulum against the plant side. You don't have to starve. Some of the gurus tell you to just drink water and fast for three days. Well, I don't think you need to. If you're just eating vegetables and a few fruits and drinking water as well, the weight will fall off you. It really will. And that's a lot more comfortable than fasting.

Here's another trick.

Let's say you get up in the morning and have some grain toast or cereal and fruit, and then have a reasonable meal for lunch - grilled fish perhaps and vegetables or salad. Then after 2 o'clock in the afternoon, only eat vegetable soup. I'll say it again - after 2 o'clock, only eat vegetable soup and a bread roll and a glass of wine if you want. Again, the weight will fall off.

You see, most people eat this giant of a meal at the end of the day and what do they do with it? They sit in a chair with it, they watch television with it, and then they take it all to bed. If you are not active, the body turns the available calories to energy stores (mostly fat) after a few hours, so the calories you took to bed have a great chance of ending up as fat. I would suggest that it may be more than reasonable to eat the larger meal in the middle of the day.

"But I just love eating," George interrupts. "I love feeding my tongue, so what I'm going to do is exercise my weight off. I'm going to get rid of my weight with exercise, all right?"

George, if you are going to try that, you should be aware of a couple of facts.

There are *3500 calories in one pound (or half a kilogram) of fat.*

And if you walk briskly for an hour, you burn around 300 calories, so you need a 12-hour walk to burn a pound or half a kilogram of fat. When you come back from your 12-hour walk, if you have a piece of pie and a beer, then you've blown the lot!

What do you think George?

"Righto, yeah ... well I'll do it harder, I'll cycle, I'll ride a bike, I'll swim."

Fine. Cycling and swimming burn 500 calories an hour so you only have to ride a bike seven hours to burn a pound of fat!

Why don't you swing the pendulum to the plant side? - it's smarter and a lot easier.

"What about running?" 1000 calories an hour. So you need three hours or more running to burn a pound of fat.

One great thing about constant and regular exercising though is that you increase your metabolic rate.

Do you know what the metabolic rate is? It is the basic rate at which you burn calories. Some people are genetically unfortunate. They walk past a fast-food outlet and put on 3-4 pounds just walking by. Other people are thinner and eat more, much more. You hate them, but it is the inherent metabolic rate they have. It's their good luck and your bad luck. Don't forget though, you can be thin and still fill your arteries with sludge.

You can increase your metabolic rate by smoking, but that's really stupid. That's why people who give up the smokes put on weight. Sure they tend to eat more, but the metabolic rate is slowing down.

If you are overweight and you smoke, it might be a good idea to trim some pounds off first and then give up smoking, because if you give up smoking first and more weight goes on, it's very hard to move the pounds. Once calories are fat, it's harder to get rid of. And don't use that as an excuse for not giving up smoking.

Exercise actually increases your metabolic rate, so not only are you burning more calories while you are exercising, you are burning more while you are at the office, while you are watching television, while you are in bed at night. It's a very good idea this exercise business.

George says, "What about sex?" George *would* say that.

Well, sex is 400 calories...

an hour.

George's wife asked me to work out two minutes ... that's 13 calories, Rosie - about a sixth of a beer!

There is another sort of sex called EMS. That's extra marital sex. 600 calories an hour! But it can kill you.

Now let's look at long-term exercise.

If you sit on your backside you burn 100 calories an hour, and if you walk you burn 300. That's 200 difference.

What if you walk briskly for half an hour each day? You would burn an extra hundred calories a day, seven days in a week - 700.

In five weeks - 3500 - that's a pound.

In 50 weeks - a lot of pounds: 10 in fact (5kg). Ten pounds, just walking briskly ... terrific...

Not much in a year, you say? Well, listen to this - those are the 10 pounds that are going to stay off.

THE THIRD THIRD OF MANAGEMENT SKILLS CONTINUED

Getting back to this stress business.

We're back to where we started, you say? You could be right. We're going around in circles.

I told you that you can learn to love pressure.

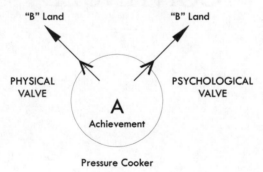

There's the pressure cooker; there's the pressure outside and here is the stress on the inside. Don't forget you can react in a positive, neutral, or negative way - it's your choice. "That's fine, but how do I become positive instead of negative?"

Right. The first thing you have to understand is this - you cannot achieve without pressure, so you need to learn to like pressure. If you want to get places and climb ladders, you need pressure, because you can't achieve without it. Makes sense? Pressure is very stimulating in bursts, but in big chronic lumps it will eventually get to you.

Now, see these little valves on the pressure cooker - these valves are what allows the whole thing to work.

When people start stewing themselves, it's because they stay in the pressure cooker eight days a week, 52 weeks a year, and it means they never get on the outside. This is where people go wrong. That's why the two valves are there. The two valves are two escapes. One is a physical valve and the other is a psychological valve. The outside of the pressure cooker is called 'B' land.

Inside is *A* for *Achievement, A* for *Type A behaviour*. Outside is *B Type behaviour* - it's the other side of you. Or maybe it's the other side of you that doesn't exist right now?

The great things about jumping out of the pressure cooker are these.

When you are on the outside, you see the problems and hassles in a different light. There is a different perspective, and quite often the solution to a problem is much clearer.

Also, when you are on the outside, you relax a little, then you begin to get excited again and you want to jump back in.

Type A maniacs cannot lie on a beach for more than a day and a half without getting agitated and excited again. "What's next?" "Where's the ball?" "What's going on now?"

You have to get out physically. Open the valve. Short term, you are allowed to stretch. Chinese employees have been stretching for decades before their cuppa - it's a little 'B' time before the tea break or coffee break.

You're allowed to take a deep breath - even without a cigarette. You're allowed to just sit there, loosen your tie or loosen your blouse, and take two or three deep breaths. Pulse rate down, blood pressure down, spasm goes ... dream a little.

Long term, you have committed one percent of your time to movement. As I said, instead of thinking fitness, think of it rather as opening the valve on the pressure cooker ... take a walk, wander around the botanical gardens and smell a rose. This is the one per cent of the time when you are lightly puffing and you feel good ... there is oxygen racing through your lungs; you're lubricating joints; you are bouncing.

It's a fabulous feeling. And you don't need to bust your guts doing it.

It is also important to open the psychological valve. There are ways to do it and you *must do* it.

Laughter is a great way to switch off. You can die laughing but you can't get sick laughing! In tough times, it is convenient that the comedies are still on television.

Even the half-hour situation comedies - watch them now and then.

"But I couldn't watch that silly stuff." Of course you could. People are embarrassed to laugh. Laugh a little, lighten up a little, get on the outside of the pressure cooker. You deserve it. Some people take themselves *so* seriously.

Try laughing at yourself ... go look in the mirror and pull a face. If you're so serious that you can't laugh at yourself, then you're in big strife.

See the funny side of things.

Relaxation techniques are very handy. Most of us disregard them, and make snide remarks....

"I don't want to lie on a bed of nails for 3 days and all that."

You don't need to lie on a bed of nails. I can even teach you a little relaxation technique - the shortest relaxation technique in the world - in seven minutes. I'll switch your body off in seven minutes. It's as simple as that.

MENTAL BONUSES

Mental bonuses are things that you look forward to, things you should be doing but probably never do.

Type A maniacs never buy a book. They don't buy a racy novel and read a chapter now and then; they don't go to movies (they haven't got time); they don't lie on beaches; they don't fish; they never walk around the gardens on a Sunday and smell the roses (they haven't got time).

Their answer?

"I'm an achiever. I'm a success, I haven't got time."

But you have got time ... that's the 'B' time ... That's the *out-of-the-pressure-cooker* time.

If you don't get out of the pressure cooker, you stew yourself. The weakest link in your chain will eventually break - hopefully a migraine rather than a heart scare.

The best mental bonus ever invented is the three-day, three times a year switch-off.

Now that's every four months ... just 3 days.

It's a total of nine days in 365 *just for you*. It might be a bit selfish but I'll tell you what, it works. No work, no home, you must get away.

"Where?"

I don't care where. Where would you like to go? Turn the clock back 10 or 20 years - where did you love to go then?

With despair, George says, "I couldn't take three days off, like I'm busy you know. I'm real busy."

If you pop a weekend into the three days, then it's only Friday you'll miss. "No, I couldn't do it."

Well give me your diary. Let's see, I've turned the pages and I'm now four months ahead. Your diary is all blank George, no Friday appointments. "Yeah, but I'll be busy in four months, it'll be full of appointments." But you're not busy now in four months are you? ... the pages are blank. Who's kidding who?

Your name might be on the front of your diary but it's not on the inside with all the VIP's.

So why isn't your name on the inside?

I'm going to write it in, all over these three blank pages, four months out - Jones, Jones and Jones. It's fantastic you know. The human brain loves looking forward to things and every time you're hassled, at least you have something out there to think about. In a few weeks I'll be doing so and so.

Do you know what? Type A maniacs never ever get everything done. There is always something to do. This technique gives you maniacs a genuine chance three times a year to clean everything up and get things done. It's a real buffer.

You get really clever with 10 days to go and start delegating. Then five days to go, you stay back late or you get to the office a couple of hours earlier to fix up those last few things. You just sweep it all away and off you go for three days, or maybe even four or five days. Then you come back and the whole world might have fallen in, but who cares? You feel good about it, and you are going to do it again in another four months.

George asks, "Just me, by myself?" Well maybe, maybe you take a friend, maybe you take your best mate (or mates), spouse, or maybe you take one of your kids (if you can remember their names), or maybe it *is* just you.

Your spouse or friend needs to understand this. So there are three types of breaks.

First there is the selfish break.

Then there is the spouse break or partner break. "What do you actually mean by that?"

I mean you and your spouse sneak away for two or three days now and then, don't you? "Just the two of us? Aw, mate, we couldn't do that." Why not? "Well, for one thing, we've got the kids you know."

So dump your kids with someone else and they'll leave theirs with you when they want to go away. A touch of reciprocation. You've got to do it.

People in business work at things, don't they? They sharpen their pencils, they make tough decisions. Relationships are tough too; you've got to work at a relationship.

"How?" Perhaps a thank-you note, a bunch of flowers, a dinner appointment. "What, with my *wife?*"

The spouse or partner break is so important. People tell me that I wouldn't know what I was talking about. Wrong. I've been married to a lovely girl for many years and we have five kids. We always sneak away four or five times a year for two or three days here and there.

Even if you travel to another country on business - if you go to Europe, you go to America, you go somewhere else - there's always somewhere nearby like an island you can sit on for a couple of days and read a book, walk on a beach, sip a cocktail.

"I couldn't do that, I've got to get home." Why? "I just have to."

No, George, you don't just have to. That's my point. You're a long time dead. Remember there are nine selfish days in the year as well as the spouse break, and then there's the third type of break - the vacation with the kids. The family break may or may not be a disaster. That depends on your attitude.

You've got to work at things.

It's interesting that many people under pressure act in a peculiar manner. The majority of people under pressure start to squeeze their brains down into what I call corridor thinking. That's where people think up and down in an enclosed space and they use maybe only 15% of the capacity of their brain power, that's all.

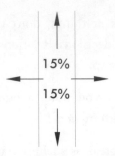

It's considered safety thinking - not very adventurous, but very conservative. I'm in the comfort zone. I'm OK. But are you OK?

It's not a bad idea to start thinking sideways sooner rather than later, because things might get even worse, and if the walls of that corridor get closer and closer and slam together, a contingency plan is your only way out. Even thinking a *little* bit sideways is allowable.

Every cloud has a silver lining.

Sideways thinking is *lateral thinking*. It's just another way of looking at things.

As soon as children think of something, they say it. Kids are brilliant at lateral thinking because it's so natural for them. We actually laugh at things kids say because we think they're funny, but kids don't think what they've said is funny - they think it's normal.

Do you know why?

Because kids' brains haven't as yet been squeezed by society, by the social rules, the corporate rules, the "you can do this", "but you can't do that". Their minds are free, not bound by the chains of conformity. They think upwards, downwards, sideways and every which way.

Then, as we grow up, we grow into moulds, and especially so when the pressure is on.

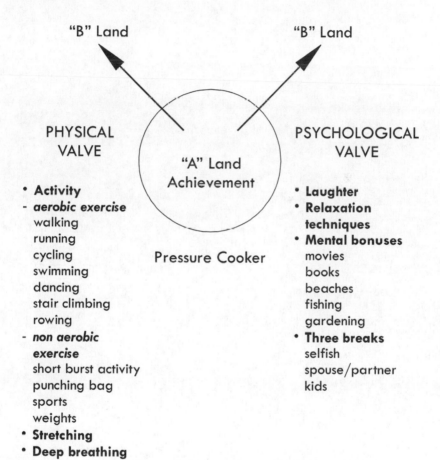

"B" Land   "B" Land

PHYSICAL   PSYCHOLOGICAL
VALVE   VALVE

"A" Land
Achievement

Pressure Cooker

- **Activity**   • **Laughter**
- *aerobic exercise*   • **Relaxation**
  walking   **techniques**
  running   • **Mental bonuses**
  cycling   movies
  swimming   books
  dancing   beaches
  stair climbing   fishing
  rowing   gardening
- *non aerobic*   • **Three breaks**
  exercise   selfish
  short burst activity   spouse/partner
  punching bag   kids
  sports
  weights
- **Stretching**
- **Deep breathing**

WORRY

George says, "But I worry a lot and have people in my business who worry all the time." So I said to him, "Do you know how to begin sorting them out?"

Take a blank page and draw a line down the middle. On this side you write CAN DO and on that side you write CAN'T DO.

Now what are you worried about?

"Umm ... the war." What war? The war's over. "Oh yeah, well, the next war, any war."

Can you do anything about it?

"I guess I could wave a banner or something ... no ... I really can't do much about it." Right, well let's put that one under CAN'T DO.

What else are you worried about?

"The mother-in-law, I worry about the mother-in-law."

Can you do anything but worry about her?

"Well, I guess I could leave home ... I guess I could ... no ... I guess not."

That's another for the CAN'T DO column.

You see you can get by with mothers-in-law, you can co-exist with them. You can co-exist with a lot of pressures.

One of the great things about the brain (which itself is like a pressure cooker) is that it has little compartments. You can put a worry (that you can't do anything about) in one of the little boxes and lock it up so it doesn't bother you except when you let it out.

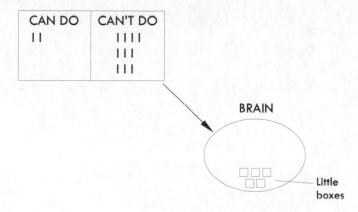

Why don't you set aside 20 minutes a day where you just worry, worry, worry about these little things and then lock them up again?

The clever people don't worry all day about these stupid things, but the worriers have the page full up in the CAN'T DO column and they have only one, two or three things in the CAN DO column.

Why are you wasting so much of your life? - it's dribbling away. You are worrying about things you cannot affect. Stick them in compartments or forget them all together. If you don't, they'll get to you and completely destroy your life. Life is for living.

What about the CAN DOs?

Do them.

Get a management plan, get an action plan going.

You can definitely help the worriers sort things out. The page with the line down the middle. Which side of the worry chart takes most of your time?

THE HORIZON

Here's the line, the horizon, which we'll call the thinking line.

Now when your business meets a hiccup or your cat dies, there is worry or grief and you get a little down. Your spirits go down, your attitude goes down ... normal human emotions ... grief, depression, anxiety, self pity ... AND YOU DIVE UNDER THE LINE.

How long are you going to stay down there if your cat dies? An hour, a day, three weeks, three months? You see most winners come up again relatively quickly; they spend 70% plus of their time thinking above the line.

Then again, I don't believe it's good to spend 100% of your thinking time way up there, because everything moves in cycles, and the contrast between down and up is rewarding.

Some people worry if they've got nothing to worry about! They would rather have a bit of pressure, a problem to work on.

The wheels are going to fall off most things some of the time, and they do, and that's good because it's the pressure, the stimulus, to turn things around.

It is frightening that your greatest asset, your mind, can turn on you and destroy you, but only if you let it.

Keep those ridiculous worries locked up in the little boxes over on the side and let them out for a breather just now and then.

If your mind does turn on you, unless you jump out of the pressure cooker and take a look at yourself from a distance, then you can go half crazy. This is a bad state of affairs.

If you go completely crazy then you end up in an asylum. This might not be so bad, because crazy people have no worries at all. It's the other people who worry about crazy people - *they're* the ones in strife.

When I was a medical student, our group spent some time observing and learning about psychiatry. We were to spend our time in an institution and on the first day I was wandering through the gardens when I came upon a patient fishing on the lawn. He was casting with his rod and reeling in the line.

I struck up a conversation with this chap and I said "Nice Day."

He said, "Yeah."

I said, "What are you doing?" He said, "Fishing."

So to humour him a little I asked, "How many have you caught today?"

He said, "You're the third!" Touché.

I HAVEN'T GOT TIME
TO RELAX

O f course you haven't.

So let's do the shortest relaxation technique in the world.

What I want to do is show you how to switch your bodies and minds off in seven minutes.

Loosen up your tie, undo your blouse or whatever (just the top button).

Take your shoes off because you need the soles of your feet on the floor so you can feel the blood flow changes.

Now just lightly close your eyes - the gentle Dreamtime eye closing.

The first part of most relaxation techniques is to concentrate on one sound, like a clock ticking, a quiet air conditioner, some music, or the sound of your own breathing. This last one is the easiest.

Next, take a couple of deep breaths. Interestingly, when you are highly pressured, you breathe with the top half of your chest, and quite quickly too. You breathe 10 to 15 to 20 times a minute because the pressure is really on and you're either pumped up or irritable, one of the two, and you breathe in a more shallow fashion. The air is going up and down, and you're not really getting much oxygen in your lungs because a lot of it is just moving up and down in the dead space of the wind pipe.

If you change the pattern and breathe with your diaphragm (that's the sheet of muscle between your chest and your stomach), like a singer, you expand the bottom of your lungs first and then the top half.

Now if you do that, you only need three or four breaths a minute instead of 10 or 15.

That gives you a lot more oxygen per breath and it is much more relaxing.

So take two or three diaphragm breaths ... nice and easy ... the pulse starts to slow down and the blood pressure begins to fall.

Let your arms relax with your hands on the thighs - soles of the feet flat on the floor - comfortable in your chair - deep breath - in we go - bottom of your lungs first - then the top of your lungs. And breathe out.....

Now those of you who are used to this technique can actually feel the pulse begin to slow down. That sensation is perhaps in your chest or the side of your head, and the heart beat is slowing down.

Take another deep breath, bottom of the lungs first, then the top ... you are starting to drift already - blood pressure is lower - spasms in the muscles are going away.

Now we wander around the body with a progressive muscular relaxation technique, and to feel the muscles relax, it is better to do the opposite thing first - contract them. That's what we are going to do. When we start, I want you to contract the left lower limb, that's your left leg. I want you to contract and tighten up your thigh muscles and the calf muscles and make a claw with your foot, as hard as you can - just like an eagle grasping a branch in high wind.

So away we go.

Tighten the thigh, tighten the calf and claw the foot. Keep it going for five seconds. That's three seconds - four seconds - five seconds, and let it go....

Relax.

Take a deep breath.

In normal circumstances you can feel an increase in temperature, an increase in warmth in the sole of your foot, as the blood vessels open out. The left leg feels heavy - heavy and relaxed.

Take a deep breath.

Now the right leg. Same again. Tighten your thigh muscles, your calf muscles and claw your foot as hard as you can ... three seconds - four seconds - five seconds, and let it go ... feel the warmth in the sole of your foot.

Deep breath.

Below the waist, your limbs are heavy and very relaxed.

Now the left arm. Squeeze your left arm into the side of your body, contract your biceps, and draw your forearm up and clench your fist as hard as you can.

Away you go ... arm into the body, contract your biceps, pull the forearm up and squeeze your fist as hard as you can ... three seconds -

four seconds - five seconds, and let it go ... hand back on thigh. Warm fingers from the increased blood flow.

Deep breath ... Relax .... Relax....

Right arm, squeeze into the chest - contract the biceps, forearm up - come on, squeeze your fist hard ... three seconds - four seconds - five seconds, and let it go. Warm fingers.

Check your legs ... heavy ... relaxed ... check your arms ... heavy ... relaxed.

Another slow deep breath.

Now the stomach. Bring your belly button (however forward it may be) and pull it back towards your spine and squeeze your stomach up, up ... come on, belly button back and squeeze your stomach ... squeeze it ... that's three seconds - four seconds - five seconds, and out she goes.

Deep breath. Relax....

Now the neck. Bring all your chins up to your teeth - like a little old granny with no teeth - chins up ... keep them up there - pull them up ... three seconds - four seconds - five seconds, and let them go....

Big breath...

Check your legs ... heavy ... check your arms ... heavy....

Stomach....

Neck ... very relaxed...

Last one. We'll do the eyes and the scalp together. Bring your hairline (wherever it may be) down to your eyebrows and scrunch your eyes up

- tighten them as hard as you can - tight, tight. You see blue, you see black, there are circles, lines ... three seconds - four seconds - five seconds, and let it go ... eyes *lightly* closed ... a slight headache ... but it's drifting off ... relax....

That usually takes three or four minutes, and then for the last three or four minutes you wander off and dream. Take your mind to a beach or a grove of trees or a windswept plain or the mountains. You choose.

Just go there and be there ... breathe easy ... come back and check everything is relaxed ... legs, arms, scalp ... back to the beach, to the mountains....

You can almost fall asleep just reading this, but it is better on tape. Get hold of my tapes and follow along as you listen.

And the great thing for all the Type A (I haven't got time) maniacs?

It only takes seven minutes.

CAVEMEN, CAVEWOMEN, CAVEPERSONS

W hat actually is the stress response?

Stress was invented way back in the dark ages, the caveman (and cavewoman) ages.

Faced with an aggressive beast they became really scared and what happened back then still happens now. The adrenal glands start surging and they pump adrenaline into the system.

When you are faced with an intense challenge, a life or death circumstance, the response is known as 'Fight or Flight'. The hair stands up on the back of your neck, the pulse rate increases, the blood rushes to the muscles which go tense, the mouth goes dry, you must make a very quick decision ... do you stay there and fight or do you run like hell?

Fight or Flight? This is the adrenaline response. It's handy stuff adrenaline because it sets you up to perform tasks that you ordinarily couldn't.

For example, women have been known to perform super human tasks, an incredible show of strength, to save their baby in danger.

Somebody screams at you in a traffic jam and you scream back and your heart is suddenly going bang, bang, bang. It would be fine if you could jump out and punch them in the face, but this is socially unacceptable.

It would be all over ... and the adrenaline response would die down. The angry animal kills you, or you kill it, or you run and you're safe ... then the adrenaline surge will go away.

But what about this life we're in?

This is *Stress City.*

Things don't die down; things stay there. There's this and there's that - we get angry, we get frustrated, there are more pressures, there are clocks to watch and deadlines to make ... the body just can't keep up.

Do you know where the adrenal glands are?

They sit on top of the kidneys. Adrenaline comes from the adrenal medulla, that's towards the centre of the little adrenal glands. But there is only so much adrenaline that can be squirted into the system.

When the acute stress response dies down and the adrenaline surge drops away, if the body is still under enormous pressure because it hasn't gotten rid of the problem, then the chronic stress response comes into play.

The adrenal cortex takes over - that's the outside piece of the little glands, and it pumps cortisone into the system. There may be 50 or more corticosteroid hormones and cortisone is one of them. You have also heard of steroids that sportspeople take to cheat. There are many different forms that can increase performance and reduce the healing time from injuries.

Cortisone can be a life-saving drug and doctors might give it to you in tablet or injection form when certain things go wrong. If you've had a kidney transplant, for example, sometimes they give you cortisone to dampen down the immune system so the new kidney is not rejected by your body. Acute asthma attacks may be treated with cortisone.

When your body starts fighting itself, as with the auto immune diseases such as rheumatoid arthritis and some tissue and skin conditions, they give you cortisone once again to stop your immune system being so aggressive.

Sure it dampens down the immune system, but you can't take excessive doses of cortisone forever because it has side effects.

Now this is amazing.

People stimulate their own adrenal glands to increase body levels of cortisone during the chronic stress responses. You are doing it to yourself day after day after day, especially if you are lousy at coping with problems.

What are the side effects of cortisone?

You retain fluid, you become bloated and put on weight; your skin starts to fall to bits because its support system is wrecked and so you get little lines, your bones can start to get soft, back pain starts to happen. You suffer from ulcers in your mouth and you can end up with ulcers in your stomach.

It's the chronic stress response - this is what we do to ourselves.

Let's say you line up for the final of the 100 metres sprint at the Olympic Games and the starter raises his gun, her gun, whoever's gun - you're on the starting blocks all pumped up ready to go ... then they decide to postpone the final until tomorrow because the wind is too strong or something like that.

Now, these finely tuned athletes are nervous: they've been building up to this; they're pumped up; they've been sitting on the toilet a few times. The adrenaline is flowing, the acute stress response - all ready to fire ... and you send them home.

What do they do? They sit around and stew.

You cancel the final the next day because of a bomb threat, and the next day because of impending storms.

This is *chronic stress.*

The body can't switch off and neither can it sit on the toilet all week.

The cortisone level starts rising, starts to chip away at the body.

Why do doctors give you cortisone? To dampen down the immune system.

What is your own cortisone doing to you? Killing the immune system, so your resistance starts to fall away and you are wide open to more colds, more influenza, more ulcers, more this, more that and, dare I say it, more cancers.

When you can't cope for long periods, that's why you get sick, because there is too much cortisone racing around your body.

That's when people start going off the rails.

They say, "Yeah well, I need more coffee, more fast foods, more cigarettes to keep me going."

Actually they don't say it, they *do* it. Eat more, drink more, smoke more.

Until something snaps.

There is an alternative. Get out of the pressure cooker into *'B Land'* - regularly. Don't argue, just do it.

I'm going to repeat a diagram and chart from around 20 pages back just in case you took no notice. This time, concentrate a little harder on the simple things that relieve the pressure and can save your life.

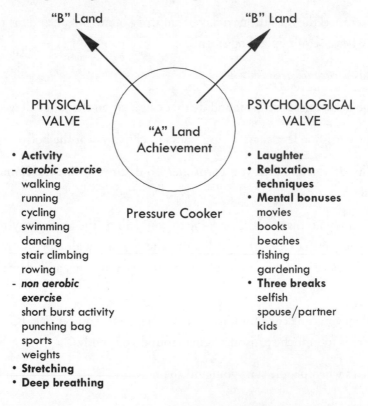

"B" Land   "B" Land

PHYSICAL VALVE

"A" Land Achievement

PSYCHOLOGICAL VALVE

Pressure Cooker

- **Activity**
- **aerobic exercise**
  walking
  running
  cycling
  swimming
  dancing
  stair climbing
  rowing
- **non aerobic exercise**
  short burst activity
  punching bag
  sports
  weights
- **Stretching**
- **Deep breathing**

- **Laughter**
- **Relaxation techniques**
- **Mental bonuses**
  movies
  books
  beaches
  fishing
  gardening
- **Three breaks**
  selfish
  spouse/partner
  kids

THE CHIEF NOURISHER IN LIFE'S FEAST

Sleep is magic stuff.

Sleep is something that seems to happen when the bacterial and other debris apparently build up in your body and the human system wants to rejuvenate itself.

We spend up to one third of our life sleeping and this can be very useful. Large chunks of our life are also spent standing in queues and worrying about things we can do nothing about. This is relatively useless.

Are America's 20 million, the UK's five million and Australia's two million insomniacs at a disadvantage? Possibly, but people who 'can't sleep' actually sleep more than they think they do, and besides, some of us get more sleep than we need.

You can't die by not sleeping, just like you can't die by holding your breath. Eventually you faint and breathe again and eventually you will fall asleep, but generally speaking the 'average' human being needs between six and 8 hours sleep each 24 hours (little kids need more) to maintain the immune system in pristine condition, to have the psychological emotions going for you, to be physically well, mentally sharp, and to have the reflex and coordination performances in top shape.

What actually is SLEEP? Well, there are two types of sleep. First there is *REM sleep* - rapid eye movement sleep. This is when your eyelids are closed, but in fact your eyes are actually darting under the eyelids and this is dream time.

The other type of sleep is *Non REM sleep*. This is the really deep sleep. It seems to be not only the quantity of sleep that is of prime importance, but the quality, the type and how long you stay there.

Normally, you lay your head down on a pillow and you drift for 10 to 15 minutes, then you plunge into the deepest Non REM sleep - deep rejuvenating sleep, and you're down there and you gradually come up through lighter stages over a period of 90 minutes or more. Next comes the first period of REM sleep for 10 or 15 minutes and then you plunge again into Non REM sleep for an hour and a half. More rejuvenation. Science has struggled to understand sleep but it seems REM sleep is also a very important and beneficial part of the sleep process. The dream time seems to lengthen as you go through the night. You might go down a third and a fourth time but the last hour or so is just pure enjoyment. This is the 'sleep-in'.

It's the bonus, the psychological bonus, it's the Sunday morning sleep-in.

Some people have a hobby called sleep. You don't really need this last bit, but some people just love it.

Right, how the hell do you get into a deep sleep?

Sleeping pills? Sleeping pills, except for occasional use, are a disaster. There are better ways. They mess up the normal physiology of the sleeping cycles.

The outstanding method is to get physically tired. Whereas mental tiredness may keep you asleep for four or five hours, genuine physical tiredness will zonk you out for eight or nine hours.

You can come home from the office absolutely stuffed, put your head on the pillow and you're out to it, but a few hours later you're awake with your brain racing around in your head and you can't get back to sleep because mental tiredness doesn't work well for the longer sleep you need.

Some people actually get by on four to four-and-a-half hours for say three or four nights, then have a crash sleep - a catch-up sleep. Some can survive like this, but some people can't and they start to get mouth ulcers and the irritability and all those things that affect their work and their relationships with other people. If you are going to play catch-ups, then two catch-up sleeps a week are needed, not just one.

By the way, definitely use the old trick of having a pad and pencil by the bed to externalise any thoughts you have that may be keeping you from sleep.

Some people are lucky, some people are unlucky, but I'll tell you again that if you get physically tired - if you put a pack on your back and take your kids for a walk through the hills - you can't *not* sleep that night. Instead of sleeping four to four-and-a-half hours, you sleep seven to nine hours of brilliant sleep. You know, most people never get genuinely, physically tired. They just don't.

Paddle a canoe for a while. "But I never paddle a canoe." That's exactly right; you never paddle a canoe. You're too cosy, too comfortable in your ways. In fact, you never do *anything!*

Interestingly, some runners go for a run to get tired but they can't because the body is used to running, so swim across a river instead, or dig holes in the garden. Use some muscles that you don't use very often. If you get physically tired at least once a week you'll have a sensational sleep ... try it.

Why do little kids sleep so well? Because as soon as the classroom door opens they run and jump and move non-stop. They get physically tired.

Why do so many adults sleep so badly? Because they sit behind desks and worry about things such as money and what other people think of them.

The old counting-the-sheep routine is not as silly as it sounds. You should be able to give your brain two simultaneous tasks that shut off the outside world. For example, if you hum, or you chant, or if you say the word "one" subconsciously over and over again, and while you are doing that, give yourself a mental task - take seven from 200, and another seven from 193, and another seven from 186 - keep going and going. Keep repeating those little things and you are blocking out the rest of the world.

It is very clever and you just drift off to sleep. You can teach yourself this technique.

Other excellent ways of relaxing the brain in readiness for a great sleep are laughing, which most people have forgotten how to do, and of course the old-time cure, sex.

The physiological aftermath of the human orgasm is the best natural sleeping pill of all. So if you can have one, even with another person (depending on availability), then that works.

Alcohol can put you to sleep quickly but it can also wake you up quickly four or five hours later. The higher the dose, and the older you are, the more problems this creates. Try two AFDs instead.

"I just get boozed mate and I drop off to sleep." Good one George.

Increasing tolerance to alcohol means that the older you become, the less well it works as a sedative, so you need more and more. If you give a little kid half a bottle of Scotch, you'll kill the little kid. If you give a teenager half a bottle of Scotch, they vomit everywhere and sleep for a couple of days. The 65-year-olds who drink half a bottle of Scotch every night, certainly go to sleep, but they are awake in three or four hours because of the dehydration and the lessening sedative effect.

Two AFDs will surely get you a better sleep than turning up the booze volume.

Another tip. If you wake up after four to four-and-a-half hours and you can't get back to sleep, and if you've tried all the tricks and half an hour later you are still awake, then get out of that environment and go out to the lounge room. A few fluffy pillows on the sofa, a blanket, a black and white movie, an old travel magazine, a novel ... this is more likely to drift you off to sleep.

And a final word on sleeping pills. As I said, they are, except for occasional use, a disaster. Maybe now and then, OK, on a trip, or to help you over a hurdle for a night or two. If you take sleeping pills for two weeks you are in strife. They lose their effectiveness. You increase the dose; you become addicted. You try to stop; you have rebound insomnia.

If there is a grief situation, if you are flying overseas, I have nothing against a quarter or half a pill. Most people take too high a dosage anyway. You usually only need a quarter of a sleeping pill to knock you out for a few hours, and make sure it's a short acting pill.

If sleeping pills have been prescribed for you, one clever way to take a pill is this ... have a natural sleep for the first four hours and if you do wake up, then just take a portion, say an eighth or a sixth of the sleeping pill, to drift you through the next three or four hours. You need a short-acting pill.

Get back to basics. Get physically tired, get your brain in neutral, or take an afternoon siesta. When you take a 15-minute siesta, that can be a good boost, but if you sleep past 15 minutes then you drop down into the deep Non REM sleep and you really need it to last an hour or so to be beneficial, otherwise you wake up half way through and you are really dopey.

The Mexicans, the Northern Italians, the Greeks (and remember Winston Churchill) - they have always used these mid-day siestas brilliantly.

The shops close after lunch because everyone takes a nap for an hour or two. And it's a great party trick, because if you have one or two hours in the middle of the day, you need less in the middle of the night!

This is a problem some old people have. They say they cannot sleep at night because they have actually slept half the day sitting in their chair. So the doctor might prescribe pills which may send them ga-ga.

Nevertheless, taking a 'cat-nap' now and then can be most beneficial as a top-up mechanism in the busy world of today.

And one last thing. Heroes who tell you they only need 4 or 5 hours of sleep a night are not heroes any more - they are outdated and fooling themselves.

It is OK to admit you have 7 or 8 hours now and besides, you feel a hell of a lot better! You think better, work better, feel better, love better, do everything better.

ABOUT SUNSHINE, VITAMINS, VEGETARIANS, & BACK PAIN

Sunshine

Sunshine is good for your body and especially good for your mind.

Do you think the anti-sun lobby has gone a bit overboard?

I'll leave it to you to decide that one, but let me tell you that sunlight elevates the mood and does good things with Vitamin D and calcium metabolism.

A decent burst of sunshine makes you feel so good, but naturally you have to be careful not to get too much, especially if you have a lighter skin tone.

Don't bake from 10 am till 2 pm, and slap some protection on your skin.

If you're concerned about spots and moles and things changing shape or colour, then go visit your skin specialist. They also have families to feed you know.

I personally think you don't need to hide in closets and run away from sunshine.

If everyone had peaches and cream complexions it would be boring, and besides, I need a few wrinkles here and there to make me look wise.

And another thing.

The research is telling us there is a chemical called melatonin which is tied up with the body clock and jet lag. If you travel across time zones, then become exposed to bright sunlight for a while, your jet lag doesn't lag so much - the body catches up faster.

And listen to this.

I have a gut feel that exposure to sunlight also slows down the ageing process and I reckon that I'm going to be proven right.

Just be careful, OK?

VITAMINS

To take or not to take additional vitamins? That is the question, a question which has no straight answer.

Conservative medical research has summarised the position by uttering statements such as this....

"At present, no strong evidence can be found to support the routine preventive use of vitamins in well-nourished people."

What is a well-nourished person? The same one who works under incredible pressure, who misses out on the morning grains and fruit, who breathes toxic fumes from the city traffic and smoke stacks, who drinks coffee all day, who eats lots of fast foods, who drinks alcohol every day, and who does all the other things that lead to exceptional 'burn-up' of water-soluble vitamins?

Vitamin C and the B group are water soluble and can't be stored in the body. They burn up or disappear via urine and sweat within 12-24 hours. So we need these every day, but we don't need fat-soluble vitamins (A and D) every day because they are stored in the body's fat supplies, and most of us have plenty of fat! Besides, taking large doses of fat-soluble vitamins can cause toxic side-effects.

Vitamins are substances which make the biochemical magic possible - producing energy and making body tissues, blood cells and hormones.

Vitamins (especially C, Betacarotene, and E) are also necessary to maintain the immune system in tip-top shape, increasing resistance against infections and cancers.

There's plenty of Vitamin C in fruits, potatoes and dark-green vegetables. Betacarotene, the Vitamin A precursor, comes in dark-green leafy vegetables and yellow fruits and vegetables. Vitamin E is found in nuts, grains, certain oils and leafy greens.

Also, the cabbage family is an important source of enzymes which may increase cancer resistance. These are the 'cruciferous vegetables'- cabbage, cauliflower, brussels sprouts, broccoli. Cruciferous means cross - the leaves of these vegetables cross each other.

Sadly, the human being cannot produce its own Vitamin C, seemingly a result of evolution. Most animals *can* still produce their own Vitamin C.

For your information, here is a list of some things which can't make their own Vitamin C.

- Human beings
- Guinea pigs

- Red-vented bulbuls
- Indian fruit bats

The difference between human beings and the other three is this: the other three eat smarter then we do; they don't live by freeways and they don't smoke cigarettes.

What I'm saying is that stressful living and breathing rotten air burn up large quantities of water soluble vitamins.

The bottom line is that go-go people who live and work in pressure-cooker environments need to eat very, very well, but usually they do just the opposite.

So added vitamins might be a help during periods of chronic stress. Some doctors prescribe vitamins to pregnant women while others say they are unnecessary (the vitamins).

You shouldn't dismiss the value of added vitamins as useless when the intake or absorption of food is less than perfect, but remember that vitamins are not the be-all and end-all of health. Vitamin pills do not have any fibre, nor do they contain enzyme systems which keep the body in fine working order and help pump up the immune system. These only come in *real* food.

Copious volumes of expensive urine may flow from vitamin freaks who eat handfuls of pills every day.

And by the way, don't overcook food or store it too long, as lots of vitamins will end up in the air.

In summary, had you asked me the question at the beginning of this chapter 10 years ago, I guess I would have said "no".

Now science is moving towards the other side of the fence. There is strong evidence to suggest that the taking of additional vitamins, especially the 'antioxidant' group such as C, E and Betacarotene, can pump up the immune system and increase resistance to various diseases, including cancers.

The antioxidant group may scavenge 'free radicals', the nasty by-products of a metabolism under pressure.

The downside is negligible, the upside appears positive, but don't overdo it and do what your Mum told you to do - eat your vegies, and lots of them.

VEGETARIANISM

I have nothing against vegetarians. Some of my best friends are vegetarians. Well, I can think of one.

They say you shouldn't eat animals because they're living and all that.

I have news for them.

Vegetables don't like being eaten either, and they're living. Besides, animals eat each other, don't they?

So what's the answer? Somehow I think we're back to the Moderation Motto.

Don't get me wrong. I'm more than three-quarters vegetarian myself.

BACK PAIN

I believe the majority of back pain can be controlled by *strengthening* the stomach muscles and by *stretching* the hamstring and associated muscles.

I cannot do justice to back pain in words, because words cannot adequately explain how to correctly achieve these goals.

There is a segment about back pain in my *Corporate Video Programs* and the associated *Work Books*.

KAROSHI

Laughter, Sex, Vegetables and Fish should be read by all Japanese executives, because Japanese people seem hell bent on killing themselves the same way Americans do, and of course the 'stress' diseases are a great way to go.

At least the Japanese are smart enough to give this a name.

KAROSHI is death from overwork.

Americans have tended to turn a blind eye to the fact that the chronic stress response is often the final precipitant that pushes people over the edge, and the rest of the so-called 'civilised' world is catching up fast.

There is a *National Council for Victims of Karoshi* in Tokyo, and they have recently published a 120- page study on the subject.

I have great admiration for the dedication of Japanese business people. I worked alongside them for some years, developing the superb resort, Hyatt Regency Coolum on Queensland's Sunshine Coast, a destination where rejuvenation outside the pressure cooker is a strong probability.

Nevertheless, if you chain yourself to your desk and refuse to go home at weekends and refuse to take regular breaks, then you might be the next victim of Karoshi.

KIDS

 My wife should write this chapter, but she's not here right now, so I'll give it a go.

GENERAL RULE NO. 1:

Kid's don't do what you tell them to do - they do what you do.

You set up their behaviour patterns for them, particularly in the first five years of their lives.

You eat mainly meats and cheeses - they think that's normal.

You eat more of the vegetables, fruits, cereals, breads, pastas - they think that's normal.

You yell and scream and treat people with no respect - they think that's normal and they yell and scream and treat people with no respect.

You laugh at life - they laugh with you.

GENERAL RULE NO. 2:

No discipline - no hope.

Be firm, but fair.

GENERAL RULE NO. 3:

Be interested in their interests - chat to them often and explain things. The two biggest problems facing kids today are exactly the same problems facing adults today.

Inactivity, and the lack of knowledge about basic foods.

If you're not active, why should they be? If you don't eat breakfast, why would they?

So they don't, and they *run on empty* until their first feed of junk food for the day, setting themselves up for disaster.

Some schools are even cutting out physical education classes. Unbelievable! Who is actually running this show?

A breast surgeon friend of mine makes another interesting point. He says inactivity and an increasing intake of fat in pre-teenage girls makes for earlier menarche - that is the beginning of the menstrual cycles. This, he says, correlates with an increased risk of breast cancer in later life.

PS: If you have more than five kids, that makes you a bigger expert than I am.

GETTING OLD

There is another disease called the ageing process. It is something we do so well in Western countries, and because we do it so well, we get old real quick.

Now, there are four things that affect your life, death and disease. The first is *'genetics'*. I have told you before, your program is already printed - it is in you. If you've chosen your folks badly, you have three other shots at it, but genetics is a big one.

Then you have *'behaviour'* - we've talked about behaviour - personality types, activity patterns, eating habits, coping skills.

Next is *'environment'*. If you live in an asbestos factory, work down a mine shaft, your family is a bunch of thieves and your mates beat up old people, then your chances are limited.

The fourth thing is called the *'psyche'*. It is *mind power*. It is the most powerful of the four without any doubt.

You can do what you want with mind power. You can either shrivel up your psyche (moan, groan, dripping nose, straight to bed, phone in sick, blame other people for your mistakes, thinking down all the time, corridor thinking, worry, worry, worry) or you can expand your psyche so big that you are IN CONTROL.

Some chief executives I deal with - they don't have heart attacks - they give them! That's called stress transference. Strong people in the mind.

If you have good genetics, maybe, just maybe, you can get by with that and that alone, but I wouldn't count on it, and besides, there is no test we can run on you to decide if you're a genetic freak or not.

I'll give you a real example of mind power.

Some people are given a diagnosis of terminal cancer - only six months to live - sorry about that. But a few of those people handed that diagnosis are still alive five and 10 years later.

It's a miracle. How come?

Certainly it's a miracle. But it was the first trigger point in that person's life that forced them to make the decision to take complete control.

Back to getting old. The process is in your hands to a large extent. Much the same as everything else in life.

And, of course, there are three types of age.

Chronological, Physiological and *Psychological.*

If we didn't have calendars and department stores that sell 'Birthday presents', then Chronological Age would be irrelevant, and the latter two ages are more closely aligned anyway.

How old do you function, and how old do you think and feel?

The greatest promoters of ageing are physical and mental disuse.

If you are a medical practitioner, I dare you to prescribe for the elderly in the following order:

1. Exercise

2. Exercise

3. Exercise

Walking, cycling, swimming, dancing, weight lifting. *Weight lifting?*

That's right, weight lifting, light weights, little and often.

4. Vegetables

5. Vegetables

6. Vegetables and then if needed

7. Drugs.

Also consider that if there is reduced absorption of nutrients, added vitamins and mineral supplements can be important.

RECYCLING

These days, recycling is the *in thing* in more ways that one.

Not just paper and glass and metals - dust off the old bicycle as well.

Did you know that cycling is by far the most energy-efficient form of transport?

That's right - less fuel energy than cars, buses or trams and less human energy than walking or running.

If the old bike is as cranky as you are, then go buy a new one with a light frame, chunky tyres and gears that allow you to do things you ordinarily couldn't do.

This is fantastic!

The energy used for cycling per passenger kilometre is only one-third of the figure for walking, one-20th of that for bus or train and a mind-boggling one-50th of that for motor car and driver.

And besides, the bicycle is clean and quiet. Not only fantastic - a revelation!

There are more than 100 million bicycles produced in the world each year, which is three times the number of cars produced, so you obviously use your bike quite a deal, don't you?

So why not? What's the excuse this time?

TYPICAL MODERN DAY SCENE

Human being jumps into motor car, drives significant distance, parks in gym car park, then pedals stationary bike.

Times are a'changing.

Cycling in a Health Club is a lot safer and more of a social event.

CRYING SHAME NO. 1

One of the great disasters of the modern-day scene is that it is usual to *double our fat content* from age 20 to 60 and this is disgusting because all this fat contains miles and miles of blood vessels and if you screw all these miles on to a system of pipes with one little old pump doing the pumping, the pressure goes up in the pipes (blood pressure) and the little old pump often gives up (heart attack, death etc).

CRYING SHAME NO. 2

Not only is it usual to double our fat content, but the other thing is even worse: we generally halve our muscle content in the same age range. We lose 6 or 7 pounds of real working muscle each decade once becoming adults, because we sit on our butts becoming 'successful', whatever that is.

And when your muscles are flabby, there is more strain on the ligaments and joints which we can easily hurt just doing the simplest things like picking up a suit case or twisting, because *we have no muscle tone.*

Everybody over the age of 40 - no, I've changed my mind - over the age of 30, should be locked in a room for five minutes a day and be directed to work out with a few light weights to regain and maintain some real muscle that pumps blood effectively to all the tissues - you look better, feel better, sleep better, love better, do everything better.

Muscles also burn more energy which keeps your weight in check more easily. Sounds good.

How many years do you do this for? Until you drop dead.

CRYING SHAME NO. 3

Loss of calcium, weak bones, brittle bones, broken hip bones, wrist bones, bent spines.

What to do?

MOVE YOUR BONES

If you put your bones in a chair for most of the time, the calcium disappears and it is *very* difficult to get it all back (like impossible) by taking pills.

If you take your bones for a walk around the block every couple of days and work out now and then, the calcium stays there.

Amazing.

THE MOST COMMON DISEASES IN THE WORLD

Depression and anxiety are the most common diseases in the world. Foundations have been established and lots of money has been raised to investigate depression.

Doctors' offices are full of people with depression and anxiety and we often forget that they are both mental and physical diseases. Tranquillisers, sedatives, anti-anxiety and anti-depressant drugs are THE most commonly prescribed medications in the whole world.

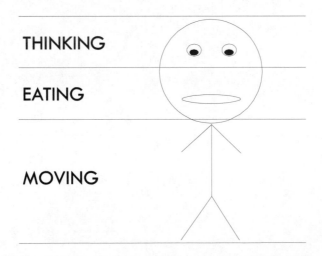

THINKING

EATING

MOVING

To begin therapy for depression and anxiety, divide the body into three pieces and start from the bottom piece, working upwards.

The chemistry in depressed peoples' cells can be improved with medication or regular exercise - your choice - but the latter is the best way to start.

This is especially so in elderly people who have promoted premature ageing via physical and mental disease.

Use it or lose it! Isn't this the same as the treatment for stress?

Exactly. All these diseases can be caused by the body deciding it doesn't like what you're doing to it. I guarantee that less than 5% of people diagnosed with serious depressive illness are fair dinkum regular exercisers.

OVERWEIGHT

Most people between 25 and 55 are overweight.

If you are under 25 and active, it is difficult to be overweight, and there are very few people past 70 who are obese. Most genuinely overweight people past 70 are dead.

If you are overweight, you are probably not a 2/3 - 1/3 eater, and for sure you get tired more easily than you should.

To realise how much extra energy you burn, try this. If you are 10 pounds overweight, tie a house brick to your belt for a couple of hours and if you are 20 pounds overweight, tie two bricks to your belt and carry them around. Not easy is it? What happens? Sore back and very tired.

Diet books make authors rich. Every diet book and every women's magazine has a different diet. There have been hundreds of them.

Some of the ones I remember well include The Seafood Diet, The All You Can Eat Diet, and The Drinking Man's Diet. This last one caught my eye. I once put a patient on the Drinking Man's Diet and in two weeks he lost 14 days.

Another favourite of mine is the Chinese Village Diet. What you eat is rice - that's it. There are no fat people in Chinese villages.

Which reminds me. Way back, I was flying an internal route in China. I was in coach class (economy). The flight attendant handed us bowls and told us to go up to first class and beg.

As you see, I'm a diet sceptic. When you go on a diet, you go *off* the diet and there is no change in attitude towards food.

Nevertheless, I have agreed to include a collection of THE BEST DIETS IN THE WORLD.

THE BEST DIETS IN THE WORLD

EATING PLANS THAT WORK

WEIGHT FOR LIFE*

If you are on the Weight For Life program, choose one of the following eating plans for the three-week duration.

Maybe a different plan for a different week, but don't chop and change from day to day.

H
ere are a few little ideas that help move your thinking towards the plant side.

When you are eating plant food you can eat a lot more food, but you are eating a lot less calories. For example, a lump of fatty meat the same *size* as a potato can contain up to four times the calories.

DR JOHN'S BANANA BUSTER
(N0. 1 PLAN)

- For effective weight loss, follow these guidelines five to seven days per week.
- For maintenance - three or four days per week.

<u>*2 Glasses of Water before every meal*</u>

BREAKFAST

Tea & Toast   Wholegrain, 2 pieces. No butter, margarine or salt.
Sliced Tomato, add pepper to taste.

OR   Small bowl of wholegrain cereal plus fresh fruit and
low fat milk.

DINNER

3 oz. fish or lean meat or chicken breast (no skin) plus minimum three vegetables (unlimited quantity) of which one is dark green, one yellow, one white.

In fact, to put a little colour in your life, choose one dark green (eg broccoli, spinach, peas, etc), one yellow (eg carrots, pumpkin) and one white (eg potato, cauliflower, cabbage). Regular brown rice (spiced if you wish) makes a great alternative to potato - not fried rice.

Make sure you're getting cruciferous vegetables most days - eg cauliflower, cabbage, broccoli, brussels sprouts.

In between times, any time you are hungry........

- Eat half a banana and drink two glasses of water.
- A reasonable maximum is eight half bananas, or four whole bananas a day.
- You can squash or mash banana on a piece of wholegrain bread if you wish (no butter or margarine).
- Keep a banana in your desk, glove box, case.

OR Eat an oat bran muffin, and drink two glasses of water.

OR A low calorie rice cake.

Avoid alcohol on banana buster days.

Tea/Coffee   Maximum three cups per day.

DR JOHN'S THREE-WEEK VFCF EATING PLAN (N0.2 PLAN)

(Vegetable/Fruits/Chicken/Fish)

- You may eat any fruits, vegetables, salads with the exception of avocado and olives.
- No added salt at the table.
- No oils. Try vinegar and/or lemon juice as dressing.
- No cooking in fat - suggest grill, broil, boil, steam or microwave. You can pan fry in a non-stick pan. A wok is a great alternative.
- White meat - eg chicken breast (skin removed before cooking) or fish. Either of these - maximum seven meals per week.
- Breakfast - fresh fruit and one or two pieces of wholegrain bread or toast (spread with banana, tomato, asparagus etc) - no butter or margarine.
- Apart from skim milk or skinny milk or low fat milk, no dairy foods, no butter (or margarine), cheese, or eggs.
- No red meats. (Veal, lamb and pork are RED meats).

FLUIDS

Tap water, soda water, mineral water - NO tonic water.

<u>*2 Glasses of Water before every meal.*</u>

- Black coffee or tea. NO sugar - sweeteners OK.
- Alcohol if you wish, but once per week only - preferably wine. Maximum three or four drinks.
- No fruit juice - eat the fruit instead.

VITAMINS

- If this is a marked departure from your normal eating habits, I suggest you take a multi-vitamin supplement every day.

SNACKS

- Fresh fruits or lightly cooked or raw vegetables. A great way to snack at the office is to pop some vegetables in a plastic bag and have this handy in your desk drawer. If you are hungry at any time, nibble on a vegetable and drink water with ice, and topped with slices of lemon.
- YOU MUST NOT GO HUNGRY

NOTES RE: THREE-WEEK EATING PLAN

BREAKFAST

Generally speaking, certain cereals, including muesli, are quite healthy, but they can be high-calorie foods and therefore better left alone during these three weeks. Many cereals contain dried fruits (high calorie) and coconut (high fat).

The grains are better eaten via a couple of pieces of wholegrain toast or bread, with some tomato, asparagus or banana. Don't use butter or margarine on the toast - the tomato etc is all you need to make it taste good.

- Don't allow gravies and sauces to be poured over a meal. If you are desperate for a little, then order it 'on the side'.
- Peppers and spices are fine - salt is not, because it can cause fluid retention.
- If you must have your coffee/ tea with milk, then make it low-fat milk.
- Fruit juice is healthy, but has far too many calories during these three weeks.
- Vegetables as snacks can be zapped in a microwave and carried around in a plastic bag in brief case, car, desk etc.

Have yourself registered as a vegetarian by your airline and each time a flight booking is made, re-affirm this directive. This way, you have an even-money chance of getting some real food in flight.

- If you cheat, then cheat on sugars, not on fats. But what's the point in cheating?

SUGGESTED MENU

2 Glasses of water before every meal.

BREAKFAST

Fruit, tea and toast with tomato.

LUNCH

- Salad or salad sandwich with or without some cottage cheese.
- Alternative is a salmon and tomato or tuna fish sandwich.

DINNER

Lightly cooked vegetables with a portion of turkey, fish, chicken breast.

DESSERTS

Fruit, with perhaps a touch of low-fat yoghurt.

- If you eat out for lunch, order grilled fish and vegetables or a salad - no sauces - lemon instead.
- No fancy appetisers - order a green salad and a wholegrain roll.

DON'T *GIVE UP - IT'S ONLY THREE WEEKS.*

Remember the fail-safe hunger stopper - vegetables in the plastic bag, or a bite of banana or an oat bran fruit muffin. The recipe in Robert Kowalski's book, *"The 8 Week Cholesterol Cure"*, is a good one.

NOTE: Any time you're hungry and not near a banana, drink two or three glasses of water.

PS. The plan is to eat this way for three weeks, then drift for a little while as suggested in the Weight For Life Video Program.

DR JOHN'S IN THE SOUP PLAN (NO. 3 PLAN)

For three weeks, or forever if you like.

2 glasses of water before every meal.

BREAKFAST

Tea and Toast

- Wholegrain, two pieces - with banana or sliced tomato (add pepper to taste). No butter, margarine or salt

OR Small bowl wholegrain cereal

Plus fresh fruit and low-fat milk.

2 glasses of water before every meal

LUNCH

Salmon or tuna fish salad

OR   3 oz fish or lean meat or chicken breast (no skin) plus vegetables or salad - with vinegar/lemon

OR   Pasta dish with a tomato-based sauce

AFTER 2 PM NOTHING MUST PASS YOUR LIPS EXCEPT

Vegetable soup - no added cheese or creams.

You can try other soups now and then, but vegetable soup works best and is best (home made is better still). If you wish, make a minestrone with as many different vegetables as you can find - add a little pasta or rice - maybe a touch of low-fat cheese.

Bread rolls - (preferably wholegrain) and one glass of wine - if you really must, but better without.

So dinner is a hearty bowl or two of soup (repeat - home made vegetable or minestrone is way ahead of the rest) and a couple of bread rolls (a very thin margarine or canola spread if you need it) and an optional glass of wine.

Late night snack - more soup.

If you're desperate, have a banana and two glasses of water.

A low-calorie rice cake is another good snack.

OK. Once a week have two or three glasses of wine - be a devil! But no beer.

DON'T FORGET - TAKE YOUR HOME-MADE VEGETABLE SOUP TO THE OFFICE IN A FLASK.

N.B. WEIGHT FOR LIFERS

Dr John's In The Soup Plan seems to be the favourite way to break a plateau period or a rising weight period.

THE SCARIEST DISEASE

During my workshop sessions, I often list a number of diseases and ask the people involved which disease is the one they *absolutely* don't want to happen to them.

Way out in front every time is cancer. Up to 30% of us are developing cancer of some type and cancer is seen as a debilitating disease which dismantles the human body and mind. It is also very tough on relatives and loved ones. What's more, depending on which statistics you believe, the death rates from cancer may not have changed much over the past few years.

In fact, in the past 10 years, the statistics show the incidence of many cancers may have actually risen. At least lung cancer incidence is dropping, except of course in the 'developing' countries where they hand out cigarettes free to school kids to get them hooked. The other good news is that science seems to be winning the battle against many childhood cancers.

Surviving cancer for five years is generally talked of in terms of a cure. Five-year survival rates have definitely improved, but the sceptics say this is mainly due to earlier detection rather than any miraculous advance in treatments - you just know you've got it longer.

And, of course, the finger is being pointed hard at those who want mass screening of populations for the likes of prostate cancer, because the simple fact is that a substantial percentage of elderly males have prostate cancer anyway.

In other words, it is there, but not life-threatening. You're probably not going to die from it.

So if you found all the early prostate cancers in the elderly and treated them aggressively, all the evidence must be carefully considered because the treatment often may be worse than the disease and the cost would be incredible.

Generally speaking, it seems that in younger people (late 40s and 50s) prostate cancer advances more rapidly and is far more dangerous and therefore more radical treatment may produce the best results.

One school of thought is that regular sex may help men reduce the risk of prostate cancer.

Males over the age of 40 also need to develop the habit of having a regular check-up. Women seem to be far more attuned to this concept for various reasons, including the fact that in the past breast cancer has been in the spotlight far more often than male problems.

Maybe we need to totally change our outlook and back pedal to the beginning.

Cancer didn't start yesterday or last week or last year. It starts way back - maybe five or so years ago. We can postulate that mitotic cells (rapidly dividing cells) happen all the time in our body and it is up to our immune system to knock out all these pre-cancerous cells daily. If our immune system is in poor working order, then these cells start to multiply until they become clinically obvious tumours sometime later.

When you study various populations around the world, it seems there are dramatic differences in the incidence of specific cancers in different countries and yet migrating populations tend to take on the cancer profiles of their new country. This means (doesn't it?) that environmental factors are more important than genetic factors in many cancers such as bowel, breast and prostate.

And as the living habits and eating habits change in a population that stays at home (such as Japan), so do the cancer profiles.

There is absolutely no doubt in my mind that the hurried, pressured, inactive, fat-filled, synthetic lifestyle thrust on us has the most to answer for.

One very credible person once said to me that you can tell how long a person will live by watching how fast they breathe. The slower they breathe, the longer they live.

Pretend you have a finite number of breaths in your lifetime and don't use them too quickly!

SLOW DOWN now and then and take some long, easy, deep breaths.

KEEP RELATIVELY ACTIVE — there is no excuse.

IF YOU SMOKE you are out of your cotton pickin' brain.

START PUMPING lots of vegetables and fruits into your system - every day that is humanly possible. Vegetables and fruits contain all the goodies (the micro nutrients) - this is where the action is. This is where all the antioxidants are and they're very, very good for your immune system.

WHAT THE HELL ARE ANTIOXIDANTS?

Antioxidants are *things* that gobble up nasties.

Things like Ernie-E™, Cecil-C™, Betty-Carotene™ and Basil-B™.

Nasties are produced by a body under pressure, a body that eats lousy food, is slobbish, inactive, worries too much, smokes, drinks lots of booze, and a body that generally cannot cope with the pressures of life.

Nasties are also produced by bodies that exercise to excess, are very intense, and maybe don't sleep too well. Being aggressive and unfriendly doesn't help either.

If you have lots of nasties wandering around inside you, they stuff up your immune system and you are then more prone to colds, flu, cancers and illness in general. Apart from that, you age faster than the calendar. Understand? You get older, quicker.

Another name for nasties is 'free radicals'. The human system actually needs a few free radicals but if there are too many, things go berserk.

This is where lots of Ernies, Cecils, Basils and Bettys come in handy. These guys also have other mates that bash the hell out of unwanted free radicals.

It is incredible how many millions of these *antioxidant things* are in vegetables and fruits.

People also swallow pills with *antioxidant things* in them, and these may help to a certain extent.

I am convinced that many of the antioxidants act in concert, like an orchestra.

If only the tuba player and the violinist show up, it doesn't sound so good, but if the whole orchestra is there, you have a top chance of a great show, especially if the conductor is there as well.

The conductor brings in concert all the enzyme systems and other micro nutrients in food that make the whole show tick. It all comes together and makes you work really well.

SO MY SUMMATION IS THIS:

While the proof is there that people who eat all the antioxidants, vitamins, minerals and enzyme systems in vegetables and fruits have less disease (especially cancer) and live longer, it is also possibly helpful to take antioxidant pills if you don't live in a perfect world, eat perfect food and have perfect habits.

Will anyone ever be able to prove that longer life is available in bottles?

I somehow doubt it, because you can't run a strict double blind trial with vitamin pills. It just doesn't work.

What's a double blind trial, did you say George?

That is where half the people take real pills, the other half sugar pills, you measure all the differences, then you swap the groups over and do it again. By the way, the guinea pigs don't know who's taking what.

The problem is this: the people who are taking the sugar pills aren't supposed to be taking the nutrients in the real pills, but those same nutrients are in food and you can't tell the people to stop eating food, now can you? So nobody knows if they're Arthur or Martha.

If you *are* going to take antioxidants in the form of pills, I have no problems with that.

If you live in a perfect unpolluted world, eat perfect food, and you handle life perfectly, you almost certainly don't need them.

But then who does all of the above?

Antioxidant therapy has an upside, and little if any downside, but remember, these pills are an adjunct, not the be-all and end-all of health. They do *not* replace good food. You cannot live on fried chicken and vitamins. And don't overdo it. More is not necessarily better because some vitamins can be toxic (poisonous) to the system.

Other supplements you might consider are the powdered extracts of fruits and vegetables which come in capsule form. These are probably closer to the full orchestra.

And if you are obsessional and can't exist without scoring points every day, try this. The scoring system is somewhat simple...

for a YES you score 1 point and for a NO you score 0 points.

"Can I cheat?" Sure George, cheat if you like, but you're fooling yourself, not me. This scorecard will tell you how you're travelling in life, how strong is your immune system; how powerful you are under pressure; how vulnerable you are in the cancer stakes.

By the way, if you smoke, don't even bother to take this test. Try walking across the road several times a day with a blindfold on instead.

Here we go...

POWERFUL PERSON RATING
(IMMUNE SYSTEM SCORECARD)

		1 point	0 points
1.	**Activity** during the last 3 days, 2 days out of 3 have you done some real exercise so that you are puffing lightly?	❏	❏
2.	**Eating** during the last 3 days, have you been eating 2/3, 1/3, or succumbed to the pressure - all bonus food and CATS?	❏	❏
3.	**Mental Bonuses** during the last 3 days, have you done something good for yourself - movie, book, gardens, dream time?	❏	❏
4.	**Laughter** during the last 3 days, have you laughed at life, at yourself?	❏	❏
5.	**Touching** do you have a support system - someone to hug, to talk with?	❏	❏
6.	**Hassles** do you have just a few hassles and handle them well, or is your life full of hassles?	❏	❏
7.	**Aggression** during the last 3 days, have you been in control, or have you blown it and lost your cool?	❏	❏
8.	**Relaxation Technique** during the last 3 days, have you taken your deep breaths, had a switch off, done a specific relaxation technique?	❏	❏
9.	**Thinking** during the last 3 days, have you had mainly positive thoughts, or negative thoughts?	❏	❏
10.	**Someone Else** during the last 3 days, have you done something nice for someone else?	❏	❏

Well, how did you go George? "About the middle, but I'll get better for sure."

If you scored 10, you're Superman or Superwoman. If you scored 1 or 2, stick to short stories, don't read any novels.

If you're a 'George' check your score each month and aim to improve.

SUPER FOODS

Is there such a thing as a super food? Browsing through magazines, one often comes across advertisements for extracts of something or other which could be 'the answer to life'.

My reading of the situation is this: Yes, there are super foods and no, there is not one particular super food. There is, as yet, no magic bullet. If you eat right across the range of these foods, you're in business - remember the concert? Every little bit helps.

These foods are in no particular order and no particular groupings. I am merely mentioning the ideas as they jump into my head.

Of course, the big rage these days is the antioxidants, and with good reason. It seems that certain foods, or what's in them, can block the chemicals that initiate cancer, and as I've mentioned before, cancer did not start last week or last month, but many years ago.

The *antioxidants* can snuff out oxygen free radicals, the nasties as we call them, and may even repair some of the cellular damage that has been done already.

It is truly amazing that ordinary fruits and vegetables can be so effective against the carcinogens (cancer causing agents).

Betacarotene, the precursor of Vitamin A or, if you like, the plant form of Vitamin A, is high on the super antioxidant list and it comes in yellow, orange and deep greens such as *carrots, apricots, peaches, rock melons, sweet potatoes* and *spinach*.

Betacarotene is a carotenoid. Carotenoids are red and yellow plant pigments and the carotenoids are bioflavinoids. This really makes your head spin.

Bioflavinoids are a group of plant substances with recognised antioxidant properties and some ability to cut down inflammation of tissues. Bioflavinoids can also be extracted from *red grapes* and *cranberries*.

Linus Pauling's old favourite *Vitamin C* is now a recognised antioxidant and of course Vitamin C is abundant in *citrus fruits, strawberries* and *pototoes*.

Vitamin E, another powerful antioxidant, is found in *nuts, grains, certain oils and leafy greens*. Is it just coincidental that heart disease really started to fire when breads became more and more refined, thus stuffing up the Vitamin E content in the grains?

Phytochemicals are a buzz and stack up well in cruciferous vegetables as well as in *soy beans, onions and citrus fruit*. The *cruciferous vegetables* are the *cabbage* family - *cabbage, cauliflower, brussels sprouts, broccoli, watercress, kale, turnips* and *bok choy* - so named because of the crucifix or cross-shaped arrangement of leaves or petals.

It seems if you eat these day after day it is very difficult to happen upon breast cancer, colon cancer and others. But don't overcook them as you may destroy the *indoles* (whatever they are) - possibly the cancer crunchers.

Tomatoes have *lycopene*, another antioxidant also found in *watermelons* and *apricots*. WOW! There is more available lycopene in cooked tomato (compared with raw) as well as tomato sauce and tomato paste.

All *green vegetables* are full of antioxidants and the darker the green the more anti it is - the darker the better. Other carcinogen blockers *(pungent preventives)* come in *allium vegetables* such as *garlic* and *onions*.

Garlic has long been considered an immune system booster - something to do with the sulphur compounds.

Soya beans are big time in the cancer prevention business, especially colon, stomach and skin. Genistein is in the bean, the curd (tofu), soya milk and soya flour. Dried and canned *beans* - chickpeas, lentils, kidney, pinto, navy, black, pink, white beans - are also on the good guys' list.

Soluble and insoluble fibre in various foods has been shown to be effective in lowering cholesterol levels (soluble fibre) and reducing the risk of colon cancer (insoluble fibre). Soluble fibre is found in fruit, rice, and oat bran; insoluble fibre in peelings, whole grains, corn and many vegetables.

As we wander around the world, the peculiarities of the eating habits of certain races are noteworthy.

The Mediterranean reliance on *mono-unsaturated fats* such as *olive oil* and *pastas* is well documented. These have a strong protective influence against heart disease and cancer.

The 'French paradox' is possibly a mystery - quite a deal of saturated fat, but a surprisingly low incidence of heart disease. Possibly not - the *red wine* may do the trick. Alcohol in moderation can raise the 'good cholesterol' fraction, and non-alcoholic chemicals like *resveratrol* may also help. This stuff also comes in *red grapes, purple grapes* and *dried raisins* that are not sun-dried.

Quercetin (what?) is also in *red wine, red and yellow onions, broccoli* and *yellow squash*. Well, stone the crows!

Japanese Green Tea is a winner. For some reason, this tea seems to have antioxidant properties. The Eskimos are heavy on the *Omega 3 oils* which seem to do everything. These oils come in cold water fish and can thin the blood, lower cholesterol, reduce inflammation and may help reduce arthritic pain and asthmatic reactions. They possibly reduce the risk of bowel cancer.

While we're on the subject of 'one thing does it all', *aspirin* is a blood thinner, an anti-inflammatory and may also reduce the bowel cancer risk. Don't ask me how; nobody really knows. Be careful taking aspirin without your doctor's advice - it can irritate your stomach and make it bleed, and can affect your kidneys.

I know I've missed out on naming lots of miracle foods you've heard about, but this is a good sampling.

Notice how none of these super goodies are in meat or cheese, or fast foods? They mainly seem to hang around plant foods. Funny about that.

Are you being overtaken by this feeling that you have a fairly good idea why heart disease and cancers are so prevalent in the Western world?

GOLF - THE NICKLAUS FACTOR

Sport is one of the very few happenings that maintains some sanity in the human race. It is also the only consistent positive in newspapers. Nothing else is - not politics, not business, not wars, not road tolls, not crime statistics. not weather.

Every day, everywhere, there are winners in sport.

It is great to play, it is great to watch and it stirs all the emotions.

I know a little about sport having been a record-holding hurdler and an international schoolboy cricketer, a lowish-handicap golfer, then a first-grade Australian Rules footballer. I have met and treated top international players from the Wide World of Sports. Jimmy Connors and John McEnroe stand out in my memory. I would not stand out in their memory.

Of all the sports at the upper competitive levels, there is no doubt that golf is the most difficult, for no other reason than it is a mind game that lasts not a few minutes or hours, but for four days.

There is no reflex action as in a moving ball sport and there is no throwing a game or set as part of the plan. To win Wimbledon you beat seven players, to win a major golf tournament, you beat around 140 players and more often than not, you beat yourself.

Many other sports demand more intense physical training, but the actual competition needs to be allotted a degree of difficulty. Mark Spitz, Ian Thorpe and Pieter Van Whatsisname swam brilliantly, but it is not difficult to swim 200 metres or 400 metres when you are that good.

Assuming I have no argument here so far, it is interesting to look at the honour board. Mr Penick, in his *Little Red Book*, says Jack Nicklaus (even though he didn't coach him) is the greatest golfer of all time, and Penick, who died just recently, saw them all.

There are four major golf tournaments in the world each year.

Nicklaus won 18 majors. Next best were Walter Hagan on 11, Ben Hogan and Gary Player with nine, then Watson, Palmer, Ballesteros, Faldo and a host of others.

The next superstar, Tiger Woods, having won all of the four majors already, has thrown the spotlight back on Nicklaus' record as he certainly has the ability to chase and match it.

On the major tournaments scoreboard, Peter Thomson is Australia's best - five majors - all British Opens. Greg Norman has won two. They say he's been unlucky finishing second eight times. Nicklaus finished second 19 times.

Nobody remembers second.

As Jack Nicklaus says, often you don't need to win coming down the stretch on the last day - just keep doing what you do well and the others lose.

It's all in the mind, the behaviour, the personality.

Behaviour under pressure.

If you are in THE ZONE, you're harder to crack.

I think *the* best was the US Masters in 1986 when Nicklaus, at age 46 (that's right, 46!), came from behind and beat the cream of the world's young golfers, the ones they said he couldn't compete against; the long hitters who were going to steal his mantle.

One for the oldies!

And one final thing - a lesson in life. Don't make lots of noise and raise the level of people's expectations. Don't tell them what you're going to do.

Just go do it!

SNIPPETS

Apprentice Priest

I ran into Bob in a shopping centre the other day with the usual, "How are things Bob?" greeting.

"Fabulous, just great," he replied. I like Bob - he makes feel good.

Bob has a philosophy that every day is a good day. When he wakes in the morning he thanks the Lord that he's alive today.

Why does Bob think that every day is a good day?

Maybe because he was trained to be a priest some time before his life took a different direction - *an apprentice priest* if you like.

I wish all those other miserable souls who moan and groan their way through life would take an apprentice priest's course for a year or two.

Life is an attitude, isn't it?

UP IN SMOKES

If you smoke, it immediately shows people you are an idiot without them having to work it out in other ways.

People say you can't prove cigarette smoking causes lung cancer. I agree with that statement. So you're going to keep smoking 10,000 cigarettes a year while you're waiting for the proof to come through, right?

***

The death column in the morning newspaper includes those who have quit smoking. It's amazing how they die in alphabetical order.

***

I laugh when pregnant women tell me they've given up smoking because they're pregnant. They care for the baby but couldn't give a stuff about themselves.

***

WAYS TO GIVE UP SMOKING OR AT LEAST CUT DOWN

Ways to give up:

1. Don't stick them in your face.

Ways to cut down:

1. Only smoke between midnight and 1.30 am.
2. Take two puffs then stub out the cigarette with your shoe. I had a patient who did this. It cost him a fortune and he ended up with cancer of the shoe.

QUOTATIONS I LIKE

"HAPPINESS IS A DECISION" - Denis Waitley

"PUT YOUR TRUST IN GOD AND GET A SIGNATURE FROM EVERYBODY ELSE" - My lawyer

"THE FUTURE BELONGS TO THOSE WHO PLAN FOR IT" - Colin Hayes

"IF YOU CANT SAY SOMETHING NICE ABOUT SOMEONE, DON'T SAY IT AT ALL" - Grandma

"WHY HAVE A SHOWER WITH A RAINCOAT ON?" — George, when asked if he wanted a cup of de-caf coffee

"80% OF GOOD LUCK IS HARD WORK" - lots of successful people

"THE PILOT GETS A LOT OF MONEY TO FLY THAT PLANE - LET *HIM* WORRY ABOUT IT" - George Burns on people who worry about flying

"CATCH THEM DOING SOMETHING RIGHT" - Ken Blanchard, *The One Minute Manager*

Ken Blanchard has made one of the best-ever statements here. You should relate it *especially* to kids. Some people seem to have kids to yell at and set bad examples in front of. Try like hell to catch them doing something right, then praise them for it. And remember, kids copy.

You smile, they smile.

"WHAT'S BEST? A PILE OF MONEY OR A PILE OF FRIENDS? IF YOU TAKE THE MONEY, AT LEAST YOU CAN RENT A FEW FRIENDS." Anonymous

MEMORIES IN PRACTICE

Back in the days when I was a family doctor, one of my partners in our general practice, Dr Bruce Reid, was an intolerable achiever.

If he scored worse than par at the first hole we had to start again. It was a local rule - his rule.

***

Myself and Dr Reynolds used to handle the obstetrics in the practice.

I got tired of it - mainly getting up at night, because it is very hard to get back to sleep after that. Also, obstetrics can be very formal - many obstetricians wear gloves and a bow tie - it's like going to an opening event.

***

Wednesday afternoons, I didn't play a lot of golf in those days. Instead, I went to the airport and wandered around. I sat in coffee shops and lounges, browsed through magazines, watched the planes take off and generally soaked up the atmosphere.

Some people hate airports and the smell of aeroplane fuel. I love airports - they're full of people with appointments and hustle and bustle. It's an attitude, it's excitement.

Later on, I used to get on a plane to nowhere, anywhere, to meet people, to get ideas. No pressure cooker, no telephones, just ideas spinning around and around.

The travel industry is aligning itself with my wishes for Type A people. Multiple short breaks are best for the manic As. There are three-day packages, five-day packages, weekend packages ... all sorts of packages. Make a quick decision and take off.

Awards: Best rejuvenation break - Hyatt Regency Coolum. Best do absolutely nothing break - Sebel Reef House, Palm Cove, just north of Cairns. Best Country Club - The Heritage Golf and Country Club, Wonga Park, Melbourne.

MORE SNIPPETS

IF YOU EAT TWO COOKED MEALS A DAY YOU'RE KIDDING YOURSELF.

Having someone to talk to is a very powerful medicine. Multiple studies show the value of a support group, a confidant, a close friend. The immune system is so much stronger - it is too real to ignore.

FOR OVERWEIGHT PEOPLE, FOOD IS A MAJOR EVENT. FOR NORMAL WEIGHT PEOPLE, FOOD IS SOMETHING YOU EAT WHEN YOU'RE HUNGRY.

To keep pace with the newest trends in consumer marketing, stress now comes in regular or lite.

How many copies of Laughter, Sex, Vegetables & Fish *have sold in India? I'm not too sure, but if you're reading this in the Bombay Library, note that breathing air in your polluted city is equal to smoking 10 cigarettes a day!*

The record weight loss for a patient of mine was 225 pounds. This guy lost 15 pounds every year for 15 years, and put the same 15 pounds back on after he'd lost it, every year for 15 years. Sounds familiar?

Ever watched the reaction of people when an announcement is made telling them their flight is delayed 40 minutes?

You'd think their son had crashed the car, the business had gone bust, and World War III had started all at once!

The anguish, the frustration, the abuse.

Who cares?

Phone through to the other end, tell them what's going on, go buy a novel or a magazine, then sit back and relax while they re-attach the plane engine.

What's the point of getting uptight?

People say, "I don't want to live until I'm 85" - but if you're 84 and feeling great, you definitely want to live until you're 85.

WHAT'S IN A WORD?

Use different words to describe your own feelings to yourself. Use *excitement* rather than *tension*. Your mind is excited - what's wrong with that?

Use *spasm* rather than *headache*. Your head's in spasm because you haven't been nice to yourself lately. It's asking you for a favour, a switch off.

VISUALISATION

BEFORE YOU GO TO PLAY GOLF OR TENNIS, TAKE TIME OUT TO WATCH A 20-MINUTE TAPE OF SOME BIG TOURNAMENT HIGHLIGHTS. VISUALISE YOURSELF DOING IT. IT PUMPS YOU UP. IT WORKS.

TITBITS

Married men live longer than single men, but single women live longer than married women.

***

The more sex women have, the less they think about it, but the more sex men have, the more they think about it.

It's a worry isn't it?

***

SERIOUSLY

NOTICE HOW SO MANY PEOPLE TAKE THEMSELVES FAR TOO SERIOUSLY?

FOR GOD'S SAKE, LIGHTEN UP A LITTLE.

TRY LAUGHING. YOU CAN'T BE ANGRY WHEN YOU'RE LAUGHING. YOU CAN DIE LAUGHING BUT YOU CAN'T GET SICK LAUGHING.

RECIPES

At the back of a book like this, you find the recipes.

This is a problem, because I don't seem to have any.

Just for the record, try these.

Breakfast

Some nice rough cereal or porridge. Chop up fresh fruit and add low fat milk or juice. Have a cup of tea if you like, and some grain toast.

Lunch

A salad sandwich or a tuna fish or salmon sandwich, or a turkey sandwich or a combination. Sometimes, a can of baked beans or a tin of sardines.

Go out for lunch now and then - grilled fish and salad, a bread roll, a glass of wine.

Dinner

A plate of lightly cooked vegetables with a portion of lean meat or chicken breast or turkey or fish.

Maybe some pasta and vegetables, olives, garlic, whatever. Even a vegetarian pizza now and then.

Or vegetable soup and another bowl of vegetable soup later on, and another one as well if you're hungry, and a bread roll.

Snacks

A banana
An oat bran fruit muffin
A can of baked beans
A tin of sardines
A hamburger once in a blue moon (with tomato)
A rice cake
Three glasses of water

Desserts

Fruit

Maybe with low-fat ice cream or yoghurt just sometimes.

That's enough recipes.

PS. And remember RICE - the forgotten food - the less refined, the better.

Several races of people have survived on rice for thousands of years, so it must work, right?

PILLS

For Worry

Two pills with one glass of water, one pill with two glasses of water or three glasses of water and throw away the pills.

For Tension

Take two pills and one brisk walk around the botanical gardens,

Take one pill and two brisk walks around the botanical gardens,

or

Take three brisk walks around the botanical gardens and throw away the pills.

If you have no botanical gardens to walk around, go plant your own. Working with your hands takes your mind off your problems.

FOR LIVER

There was a little old lady who took liver pills. She took so many liver pills that when she died they had to beat her liver to death with a stick.

TIME

If you can't put aside a little time now for some recreation and exercise, make sure you put aside a lot of time later for illness.

STRESS - THE COST

There is no point in telling you in dollar terms the quantum cost of stress to our community (tax payers).

The reason I'm not going to nominate the actual cost in millions of dollars is that next month the number will be wrong, simply because the payouts are escalating like crazy.

And the reasons?

1. THE SYSTEM ALLOWS IT

Is that right or wrong? No comment.

RSI is changing its face, from Repetition Strain Injury to Really Stressed Individuals.

2. LIFE HAS BECOME TOO COMPLICATED

You can see it with the kids - the pressure is on right from the start. Instead of playing ball, we play with plastic computers and munch plastic food.

3. THE ACHIEVEMENT PROCESS IS DIFFERENT

In times gone by, satisfaction for many was easier. Today, we chase the elusive something harder and harder. And if we get there, are we satisfied?

4. MANY YEARS AGO STRESS WAS NOT A WORD.

Before stress was a word we only had problems.

If we had problems, we would work our way through them and get on with life. Nowadays, if we have problems, it is called stress. We put in a claim, slap a law suit on someone and line up for counselling.

STRESS - THE PROCESS

Pressure is out there. Stress is in here.

If we like pressure, we do good.

If we *perceive* that we don't like pressure, we have two ways to go.

Either walk away from it or do bad.

Of course we can change the perception if we want to - think differently, handle it better, turn it around - but usually we don't want to, or don't know how.

Stress doesn't need to make people sick.

Is it the system's fault or is it the individual's fault? Both, but more so the latter.

STRESS - THE ANSWER

1. Divide the human body into three pieces

    (i) Above the nose

    (ii) Between the nose and the neck

    (iii) Below the neck

    The top bit is for THINKING, the middle for EATING and the lowest part is for MOVING.

If (ii) and (iii) aren't working very well (or maybe not working at all), (i) is in huge trouble.

If all three pieces are in good working order, the ability to handle pressure dramatically escalates and negative stress is minimised.

2. Give everyone a copy of Dr John's book - it works.

3. Set a seminar or workshop date with Dr John for your people - it works.

Now that you've read the book....

You should see the movie, Dr John Tickell's Video Program titled, *Stress and Success Beyond 2000.*

Learn how to love pressure and turn stress into success.

"Great video," says George, "Good for the business, good for the kids. Perfect for management training in companies and for schools, hospitals and homes."

See the following page to order Dr John Tickell's video program.

To contact Dr John Tickell
for speaking engagements and corporate presentations :
Email: drjohntickell@drjohntickell.com

To order books, videos, audio tapes, DVD's, CD's,
newsletters and for general information on health, stress
and nutrition :

Website : www.drjohntickell.com